AN AMERICAN HEALTH PLAN

An American Health Plan

*An insider exposes damaged
care and denounces Obamacare*

by Corinne M. DiBlasi, Ed.D., LPC

ISBN 13:978-1456477554

ISBN 10:1456477552

Printed in the United States of America

Dedication

To Karen Wenger who nursed me when I was spiraling downward with weekly spiritual gifts of prayer and listening. To St. Elizabeth's Church, and the wonderful staff who listened to me and knew I needed spiritual support more than counseling. To the community of Stephen's Ministers, a program dedicated to helping parishioners going through hard times.

TABLE OF CONTENTS

PREFACE

At first I wrote this book because of my mind opening experiences as a care manager in the so called managed care system. Next, I wrote out of my anger toward the current managed care system's inflexibility. But then I wrote because I was unemployed, uninsured and sick, and discovered how to get cheaper healthcare without managed care. I kept writing because our nation was debating a revolutionary health care bill. And finally, I wrote because a new health care law passed in March 2010 and it portends to be the answer to all our country's health care problems yet it repeats the ills of managed care!

With our nation's unemployment rising and health care costs climbing, many suspect the new law is not the panacea that some tout it to be. Fear abounds as we anticipate some of it's consequences. Popular politicians promise to have it repealed. It is time for us to open another debate about affordable health care and how to make that happen. It has to fit America, in all its uniqueness. It cannot be imported from somewhere else. It has to deliver quantity and quality care, not reduced care or watered down care or limited care. It has to be available to all who want it.

When I became unemployed and sick at the same time, which should not surprise those who understand the closely related mind, body and spirit of the human species, I panicked. Then I got on the internet to search for information about my symptoms. I procrastinated, became anxious and felt alone and hopeless. Fortunately, I had some retirement savings to tap into. So I set about to determine what illness I had and get it treated. Well, treatments are aplenty, I learned. But what was the illness? I needed to become a detective, or to find some doctor-detective, or maybe even a team of doctor-detectives. Not only was I not up for the task, but I learned that the many doctors I visited were not either. Here is when I came to the conclusion that medical care has declined in quality. I went from a general practitioner to an ear, nose and throat specialist to a cardiologist to a pulmonologist.   Each visit was a whopping $250 plus.   Still, none could diagnose my problem without expensive tests. So I went ahead and had the costly test which rendered a diagnosis of a rare lung disease, only to be told that this was probably not my problem! More tests were suggested under the vague description of auto-immune conditions. The pulmonologist asks if the ear, nose and throat specialist did a CAT Scan of my head... Well, no -- was he supposed to? The games went on for almost nine months before a general practitioner suggested I accept treatment for the symptoms since I may never know what the heck caused my rare lung disease and it is the only diagnosis I had to go on. Ten thousand dollars later, I found some alleviation of my symptoms from a rare lung disease that is "probably not" my problem! Does this sound like an efficient system? It did not to me either.

After returning to the field of education as a college professor, I was finally among the fortunate who have employer funded health care. My symptoms are under control, thank God. Then, several motor vehicle accidents alert me that my eye sight was deteriorating. This was diagnosed as cataracts. Should cataract surgery be covered by health insurance? BCBS does not believe so.... unless I pay my $2000 "deductible". The fact that I did not yet meet the deductible by the end of the year presumes that my health was good and I did not need services. Instead of being rewarded, I am saddled with the $2000 penalty. No exaggeration, I read my policy at least five times and spoke to upwards of ten "representatives" from the BS plan before learning that I must use an "in network" doctor (150 miles outside my town) and that the doctor will be covered but the use of his clinic will not be!

None of the reps seemed to agree with me that blindness was a serious condition . The specific term "cataract" did not appear in their policy. There were "eye implants" and "cornea transplants" but no cataract. After going round and round with these folks, I knew I had to have this surgery regardless of whether it was going to be covered or not. Though there was a doctor with a better reputation, he was "out of network" so I had surgery by the in-network doctor for an astounding $2500 per eye with a $50 co-pay per eye and an additional $800 for the use of the clinic. Total out of pocket cost to me was $2900 for this procedure and $1200 for my portion of this year's policy term, or $4100. As if that was not enough, one year later I developed what is known as a "secondary cataract". Bottom line: I can't see! Is this procedure covered by the BS, I mean BCBS plan? Not! This one cost me $1500 out of pocket and a 300 mile round trip.

Now, I may be somewhat particular, but I would have preferred to avoid the hassling representatives altogether and go to the doctor of my choice after interviewing the best of them. It appeared to me that the cost of surgery was jacked up by the provider (there were beaucoup patients lined up in portable beds for the very same surgery I was having), and the vagueness in the policy allowed the managed care company to extort it's profit. Many of you have similar stories that we can horrify each other with.

In this book, you will hear about a very broken health care system managed by "damaged care", and a not so new overhauled health care system from an Insider. The first has been spoiled by too many interest groups and their greedy ambitions and federal involvement. The second is borne from tweaking the first, gleaning what is good and dumping the warts. <u>An American Health Plan</u> is a hearty soup of ingredients that fit in with our culture, our times, our needs and our expectations for excellence.

Bon Appetite!

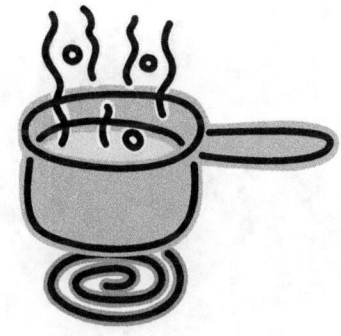

AN AMERICAN HEALTH PLAN

PART I

MANAGED CARE=DAMAGED CARE

While Americans clamor about the exorbitant price of health care, both medical and behavioral, managed care blends into the landscape like an innocent bystander, an elephant in the living room of America. This despite the "managed care backlash" of the last decade. We seem to have forgotten the function of these corporate giants with the misnomer "Managed Care"; they were intended to hold down the cost of health care. They did at one time, before they were beleaguered by government interference. Currently, managed care no longer works, and the way they are structured they probably never will. In addition to the failure to hold down costs, quality of care has declined as well. Now, Managed Care is Damaged Care.

Why are managed care companies failing to manage health care costs? If you think that managed care is strangled by over regulation, you'd be right. That said, if you think that managed care is suffering from lack of regulation, you'd also be right. The truth from this insider is that managed care is plagued by both over regulation and under regulation. Service to patients is over regulated while management of health care costs is under regulated. Defenders of managed care ask: "How much worse would it be without managed care?" No one knows the answer to this but what is more relevant is that managed care can and should be doing much better than it is. Bottom line: managed care is not managing health care costs, is enabling the decline of quality of care, and leaves under-served policyholders disappointed and angry with almost every contact. Policy makers are missing the real leak in the boat, applying temporary patches that serve to worsen the situation and cost tax payers even more. Where is our outrage? Though we agree that this industry has become a three ring circus failure, we continue to live with it and support it! The alternatives to some policymakers is this and that new policy while still tolerating the massive mess that is damaged care. Why everything imaginable has been proposed except to dismantle and eliminate managed care!

Spending Up, Quality Down

According to the most recent report released in September 2010, (Income, Poverty and Health Insurance Coverage in the United States: 2009, pp 30-34), 63.9 percent of the population was covered by private health insurance and 55.8 percent of that population was covered by employer based private insurance. This is the lowest number since 1987. In the same report, 30.6 percent were covered by government funded health insurance. This is the highest rate since 1984 The government funded programs are almost equally divided between Medicaid and Medicare with a very small percentage going to military health care coverage. The uninsured population has grown steadily and as of this report stands at 16,7 percent. ("Data Points: Health Insurance Coverage...", US News & World Report, 2008).

While private and public health insurance initially improved the access we have to care, this author wonders, at what cost? Premiums, deductibles and co-pays are rising rapidly while services become more limited. The inefficiency of managed care is recognized in much of the literature review on this topic. Readers will discover some of these indictments and some of the literature that attempts to explain the rise in health care costs.

For example, Christine Cadena describes the failure of managed care as "...an overwhelming imbalance of profits from premiums, versus claim payments". (Cadena, 2008, p 1)

But Thorpe (2005) attributes the rise in cost to a rise in the number of medical conditions treated. Thorpe contends that more and better treatments have been developed for more diseases. For instance, treatment for back problems has risen from "4.6% to 8.1%" and diabetes treatment has risen from "2.4% to 4%" (Thorpe, 2005, p 1436-1445) thanks to new innovations in treatment.

Thorpe's report makes skyrocketing costs sound like a good thing. Others suggest that more people are receiving more treatments for more diseases because of the access to internet based information on health risk factors and providers' backgrounds and ratings. This suggests that consumers know more today about their conditions and the doctors who treat them. (Lagoe, Aspling & Westert. 2005). Therefore, informed consumerism accounts for the rising costs.

In addition, State Coverage Initiatives (2008) reports that the increased cost of healthcare is due in part to "...an increase in the intensity of services, the availability of more expensive drugs and technological services, the aging population and rising administrative costs".(p1)

All this said about improved care, more intense treatments, more informed consumers, better treatment as the cause of the climbing costs of health care, it remains the responsibility of the managed care companies to manage these costs. While this author agrees that all of the reasons mentioned play a part in the increased cost of health care, but increased premiums and co-pays, and restricted care does not seem to compensate for the higher costs.

Consequences

One consequence of the skyrocketing cost of health care is that fewer people can afford health care plans. Besides the cost of premiums, co-pays and deductibles, and the many limitations in so called "covered" conditions, the non coverage of other conditions means that these conditions worsen and require more intense and more expensive treatment.

"The high cost of health insurance is consistently the most commonly cited reason for why employers do not offer coverage and why individuals do not enroll when offered coverage. Average annual premiums in 2008 were $4,704 for single coverage and $12,680 for family coverage."
(Why Are People Uninsured?, 2008, p1)
As a Board Member of a local private school, the author has been involved in deep discussions over the burden of hiring a new employee due to the regulation that health care must be offered. The decision to hire was unanimously voted down.

As people lose employment in times of economic downturn, incomes fall and health insurance is lost. Purchasing individual health care is terribly expensive and private companies are allowed to deny coverage for pre existing conditions. Between 1999 and 2008, the cost of health insurance premiums have risen 119 percent, while wages have only grown 34 percent! (State's role in cost containment, 2008)

COBRA, an extended policy from a previous employer, also involves even high premiums. But both sick and healthy folks who are unemployed are usually unable to pay these higher fees. Our previous system does not help this population at all though logic supports that these are the very individuals who need to maintain good health to continue with job search activities. It seems illogical to this author that health care should be connected to one's job at all. The new law addresses this issue by making health care "portable". This is a good thing.

Though health care will be portable, it may still be unaffordable! It is also likely that when more of the population loses health care coverage due to job loss, enrollment in Medicaid will increase. Even with low unemployment levels, Medicaid enrollment has grown by nearly one-third since the beginning of 2001, covering many people who would have otherwise been uninsured. Medicaid enrollment increases may contribute to more fraud and waste through mismanagement under a massive bureaucracy such as the government. This adds to the economic burdens of the taxpayers. After all history does repeat itself.

(Who's Uninsured?, 2008)

In short, the giant entity, *damaged care*, designed to reign in the high cost of medical and behavioral health care and improve the quality of that care now itself needs to be reigned in so that more citizens can afford it. But the many attempts to discipline this unruly monster we call "managed care" are short-sighted and unproductive, contribute little to quality of care and may create a breeding ground for rationing and unethical practices. These "adjustments" have always come in the form of new regulations—obstacles to efficient performance. If we fail to correct the mammoth problem that managed care has become, it may be suggested that it be scrapped altogether and replaced with socialized medicine, which does not have a good track record when tried in other countries. This would amount to "throwing the baby out with the bath water". Is Obamacare the fulfillment of this replacement or more of the same "damaged care" model?

Managed Car Care?

Don't misunderstand me; I am a proponent of managed care. In fact, I would like to see managed care for cars and many other commodities and services. Imagine this: Your car is purchased through a car dealer who can also sell you a car care policy (like a warranty or an insurance policy) for which you pay a modest premium. When your car is "ill", you return it in to the same independent car dealership for a diagnosis, prescription and quote. To avoid a conflict of interests the car dealer does not do repairs; instead there are specialists, like "service providers" who do this work. The owner may now bring this "diagnosis" to various repair shops who bid for the work on the vehicle. This concept is attractive to both consumers and policymakers. It certainly would cut back on needless work being done, reduce the cost of the work being done, and eliminate corrupt car repair shops that prey on the poor car owners who may know little about cars. If this principle is applied to the current system of health care as we now know it, there is clearly something missing; there is no "independent" entity who can diagnose and prescribe or recommend treatment. In fact, the managed care company has a vested interest in saving money to make a profit, not in making accurate diagnoses and coordinating services to policyholders. The managed care company has already made a deal with the providers of the services, or, as they say in politics, they are "in bed with them". Independence and objectivity are lost. Another missing element in the author's Managed Car Care policy is the huge bureaucratic waste so typical of today's managed care. Local management of services would improve delivery considerably. As for Managed Car Care, I do not believe this is a far fetched idea; recently, the author has been hearing about a car repair company offering just this type of policy with a specific list of parts and services that will be "covered" and eligible for replacement.

PART I CHAP 1

MANAGED CARE

All Nuts No Bolts

In the most typical model, insurance companies calculate to make a profit after paying the managed care company fee. The managed care company makes a profit because they deny or under treat illnesses in as many cases as possible. Managed care companies have been in place about two decades now and since their arrival, they have been evolving. Legislation, market demand, delivery systems and types of utilization are always changing. This author has been researching the profit trail, and is still unsuccessful in "following the money". But a multitude of questions arise as I make my way through the mountains of paper to understand how it all works. As consumers, we know where our money goes, so it was puzzling to me why I could not get to the bottom of it all. We know for example, we pay a yearly premium and most of us pay co-pays when we access services, the providers have to get paid, the insurance companies and MBHOs are each making profits and paying their CEOs and employers. But who gets what and why do consumers get the short end of the stick?! (Kongstvedt, 2007).

Continuing with the first model, the payment to the managed care company from the insurance company is based on research and statistics of common medical and behavioral (mental) maladies that typical humans will suffer in a typical life span. The treatments for these conditions are called "protocols", which are also based on research and statistics of what works and what does not. For example, the protocol for treating high cholesterol is cholesterol lowering drugs and blood tests twice per year along with diet and exercise. The protocol for treating depression is individual therapy with psychiatrist prescribed anti-depressants. Information about the prevalence of these conditions and their protocols are easily accessed to create a database that informs decision making in managed care and health insurance companies.

A disturbing collusion emerges: In the most common model, the insurance company has hired the managed care company for a fee along with a list of services covered and a range of costs for each service. In another model, the insurance company acts as its own managed care company. Examples of this model are Cigna, formerly known as Cigna Behavioral Health. Either way, it is simply nutty to think that the folks with the pocketbook strings should be the ones making treatment decisions!

The managed care company is a "double dipper", the ultimate "middle man" between the insurance company and the policyholder, and again, between the insurance company and the providers. Their *stated* goal is to connect the policyholder with the appropriate services needed: their mission is to keep those costs down. This seems noble and logical.   But before that can happen, all three entities involved want to make a *profit* from you, the policyholder-- who pays the ultimate tab. It's all very underhanded, or, as we like to say in the mental health field, "gamey", because no one really knows where the money is going. Your insurance company advertises that their priority is serving their policyholders. We are all familiar with the warm and fuzzy advertisements showing actors in wheelchairs who swear they would be dead without the caring services of Aetna, Cigna, Blue Cross, Humana, etc. The providers, such as the doctors, clinics and hospitals make the same claims. But the managed care company is not even listed in the phone book!   And the insurance company diverts your questions to the managed care company. When job searching and researching for this book, even internet searches seemed to play "hide and seek" with the secret little entities known as managed care companies. Do you know the name of *your* managed care company? Who is the CEO? It's just all very stealth...

This is for sure: The managed care companies, because of their symbiotic relationship with the providers, can lower their pay-outs to the providers who then may water down or limit their services. In the industry they call this "capitation". Conjures up some strange images, doesn't it?... With money passing from hands to hands you can bet there is waste, inefficiency and opportunities for fraud. You, the policyholder, are at the mercy of these vague entities all vying for the gold, the gold being your hard earned income.

Those receiving services are generally not aware that the original cost of the care is different from the resulting "contracted" cost. What would the cost of the actual services be without the dance among the insurance company, service provider and the managed care company? This author's own experiences as an uninsured consumer during 2005 can attest to lower costs when providers are paid directly. (See Analogue for details) Many providers give discounts for direct payments and cash payments. Obviously they are fed up with dealing with the managed care bureaucracy as well and they have found the discounted costs are worth it to them.

In summary, the consumer chooses or is given (by an employer) an insurance policy from an insurance company such as Aetna, Blue Cross Blue Shield, Cigna, Humana, Pacific Life,

UBH (name your poison), at some shared cost to you. This is your *premium* or your share of the premium if the employer pays some of it.   Many insurance companies do not want to manage their own policies and respective policyholders themselves.   It can get rather unsavory and the insurance company seeks clean image so they can continue to make impressive commercials and sell many other products.   In addition, management requires employees with specialized training to manage cases, policies and recommend providers. Instead, the insurance company hires a *managed care* company to orchestrate the policy, the policyholders and the service providers.   The insurance company gets to set the policyholder up with a *policy* (otherwise known as a legal piece of gobbledygook) that only the insurance company employees can completely understand, and then they turn you over to the managed care company. Like being fed to some insatiable and ferocious animal... The managed care employees are also well versed in the so called "policy", the various illnesses, the protocols and services, so at any given time you may be informed that you are *not covered* for the services you seek and/or need. (Do not hesitate to negotiate rates by appearing to know any of the esoteric "rules" in the policy, threatening to sue, or making a report to the State Board of Insurance!).

After they have gathered your information, you are informed that what you have is some esoteric illness pulled from the DSM IV (the Bible of mental conditions discussed later in this section) and can be "serviced" or "treated" by going to such and so "provider" who specializes in such and so. (Sounds like you are a carpet or something!) The providers are the specialists, clinics, hospitals, doctors, therapists, rehab centers, residential treatment programs, who will fix you up after taking your "co-pay" and deriving the rest of the cost of treatment from your benevolent insurance company or the managed care company.

These providers, as stated earlier, are also part of the scheme in that they have agreed to keep their prices within the acceptable amount already agreed to by your managed care company. (called "capitation" as stated earlier). In return, the providers expect the managed care company to refer patients to them. Volume is profit. None of these partners are working on quality of care, or if they are, it becomes obscured by a huge bureaucracy of entities, subdivisions, subsidiaries and "carve outs" .("carve-out" explained in the next section).

It appears that while taxpayers tolerate diminished quality and increased costs, others continue to line their pockets without impunity. As early as 1999 it was recognized by Liberman and Rotarius that managed care has a propensity to contract with providers who will agree to accept lower rates. They write,

"....managed care is...under scrutiny and criticism for its own hubris and its failure to serve the best interests of patients, for example, ...paying bonuses to physician administrators based on the denial of needed specialist services; and the decline of acute care referrals". (Liberman & Rotarius, 1999, p 50-57) Does anyone believe that salaries for CEOs and employees of managed care and insurance companies have declined in kind?

PART I CHAP 2

MANAGED CARE

Paradigm to Parasite

Once a terrifically creative concept which revolutionized health care delivery, managed care has more recently succumbed to over regulation, bureaucracy and greed- and yes, politics too. Don't get me wrong: I am still, as stated earlier, a proponent of managed care... for less personal goods and services! But this poorly planned baby has turned into an undisciplined teenage monster that not only drains both the recipients and the providers of the health care it was designed to facilitate, it has also provided opportunities for corruption, and now demands it's own bottom line be met *first*. Quality of care is down and cost of care is up. If you were thinking that this is why a "single payer" system would be better, look at the *great success* of Medicaid and Medicare...NOT! Medicaid horror stories abound. And since they have hooked up with Damaged Care, Medicaid can now claim double failure! As models of bureaucratic waste and inefficiency the team of Medicaid and managed care is doomed.

Deep Tentacles

The growth of MBHOs over the past two plus decades is significant. In 1997 just twelve of these MBHOs covered eighty five percent of the MBHO market. (Taub, 1998) In 2001, MBHOs more than doubled in number. (Office of Health Care Systems & Financing, 2001). While in 2008 there were 34 MBHOs. (NCQAs MBHO Report Card, 2008)

Considering that half of the plans in the 2001 list have disappeared, this is incredible growth. For example, Optum Health Behavioral Solutions did not even exist in 2001, yet they currently cover the largest population of policyholders of all the MBHOs in business at this time, forty three million lives. (American Psychiatric Association, 2008) A close second to Optum Health is Magellan with over forty two million lives. The remainder of the MBHOs each carry under twenty five million lives. (Taub, 1999)

Carve Outs & Cut Ups

The specific managed care this author has had experience with is the even more shrouded and mysterious world of managed *behavioral* health care, separate from *medical* health care. Bet you didn't know these services were managed separately and you are still looking in the telephone directory.

In general, Managed Care Organizations (MCOs) cover services related to physical health and Managed Behavioral Healthcare Organizations (MBHOs) cover behavioral health care (mental and emotional health). There are cases of "dual origin" such as dementia, and alcohol withdrawal which may be considered medical conditions, but which have symptoms typical of mental illnesses such as psychosis. Dementia is often treated in a psychiatric facility with psychotropic medicines by mental health staff, but may also appear in medical emergency rooms. Medical care and behavioral care are separate services, separate policies and separately managed. This additional mental health coverage is often called a "carve out". Carve outs are likely to result in an increase of cooks spoiling the brew. Finch, Campbell and Harbin (2006) write:

"The lack of coordination and integration among managed care vendors (MCOs, MBHOs EAPs) ..." and the rest of the alphabet soup... "has created significant quality and accountability problems". (p 6)

Frank and Garfield (2007) report from Harvard University that carve outs

> "have exacerbated existing difficulties or created new problems" because, "They are based on the economic principles of economies of specialization...of scale, price negotiation, and selection". As such, they have lowered costs, "but", the authors contend, "results on their impact on quality of care are mixed." (p 1)

Among the differences between medical and behavioral health care, perhaps the major difference is the policyholder population. A smaller portion of employed individuals suffer with mental problems compared with physical problems. But, few seriously mentally ill ("SMI") can hold a full time job down, jeopardizing their membership in a private health care plan. Many persons with less severe mental illnesses are unaware of their own conditions or are unwilling to discuss them with anyone. Mental or behavioral healthcare is not as available as medical healthcare, although some progress has been made in the legislature for "parity" laws (equal access to behavioral health care). Still, not all states have these laws, and the ones that do have found that mental health comes with its own set of management problems. "Access to specialty mental healthcare services is constrained due to a benefit design that features high co pays, visit limits, and utililization management". (Finch, Campbell & Harbin, 2006, Slide 16 #9)

These constraints simply intimidate policyholders with mental health issues from utilizing mental health services. This results in high use of the general medical system and high use of medicines without the benefit of other psycho-social interventions and even substance abuse to alleviate the symptoms. In addition, Psychiatrists are few and far between, and the ones employed by MBHOs are underpaid and often marginalized. (Mulligan, 2002)

If it were not enough that we have these unmanageable bureaucracies with little accountability and dwindling accessibility, here comes even more profound fracturing of the system. Despite the public's confusion, MBHOs love the word *"subsidiary"*. For example, Magellan Behavioral Health is a division of Magellan Health Services and other Magellan associated companies include Green Spring Health Services, Human Affairs International, Merit Behavioral Care and CMG Health. (Taub, 1999)

And Optum Health is a subsidiary of UBH, itself a subsidiary of UHG or United Health Group. Ironically, in 2006 UBH reported in an article about its new program, "Life Solutions", that "The fragmentation of the current health care system does not adequately meet the needs of patients with chronic illnesses and psychiatric disorders". You think? (Open Minds, 2006, p 1)

Is it any wonder that accessing services is a hassle for many? It often takes a barrage of questions about your employer your various code numbers, your birth date and social security number and so on before you can be identified. The impersonal nature of the contact with the managed care company is inconsistent with the nature of the very personal problems presented! Why, they barely know who *they* are! Now the policyholder bears the added confusion of whether to call the MCO or the MBHO, the "sister company" of the subsidiary or "corporate" and the "division" of the "branch" one is speaking with! If one is calling *for* a policyholder who needs help, the caller needs to ascertain what a grandparent, parent or child is suffering from to begin with. Various conditions have the same symptoms such as dementia, Alzheimer's and alcohol withdrawal. Often it is just a lot easier to rush the patient to the ER and let them figure it all out. But such is the reality of the monster before us.

All those *cooks*, (I can assure you as I have been there), receive paychecks from some company name *they* don't even recognize! It's just more of the stinking *brew* the author speaks of. Managed Behavioral Health Care Organization, MBHO, is a very confusing business for the general public; there isn't much transparency. We follow procedures like "sheeplings" (from Michael Savage, 2002) because it is nearly impossible to hold this vaguely defined entity to any accountability. Lawyer, Sara Rosenbaum (2003) writes about the liability surrounding managed care corporations and MBHOs which experience financial failure. Insurance companies who experience failure may *not* file for bankruptcy; their focus is on saving the policyholders' rights. But, Rosenbaum explains, the "hybrid nature of managed care" makes it difficult to deny these companies the *right to bankruptcy*. (Rosenbaum, 2003, p 1-4)

Bankruptcy is devastating to policyholders. The author was employed by Magellan when they declared bankruptcy; the focus is on saving and restructuring the company, not guaranteeing members continued or quality coverage or insuring their rights. In bankruptcy (euphemism: "restructuring"), members can be dropped, services can be cut off, provider contracts can be terminated and chaos may rule for consumers. But if the managed care company is *working for* the insurance company, should they be allowed to claim bankruptcy? The laws are unclear because the industry itself is unclear. As it stands now, the MCOs and MBHOs get to put their own goals ($) ahead of the policyholders, thanks to "an enormous variation in entity type" (Rosenbaum, 2003, p 1-4). They can limit covered services or include all services; they can contract with specific providers or a more comprehensive list of providers; they can cover mental health conditions or only medical conditions; they can be the managed care company and the insurance carrier all in one. Some examples of the "all in one" models are Cigna , Aetna, Pacific Life. MBHOs can assume risk (do not sell insurance) or not (non-risk entities like Magellan). This is not only confusing, it's a recipe for disaster.

Separate and NOT equal...

The separation in management of behavioral health care coverage and medical health care coverage, has some advantages and disadvantages. An advantage to separation of the two lies in the very nature of the mental health population. They are prone to overlook their own need for help. The very symptoms of depression in fact, cloud the thought processes of sufferers who then become non compliant with their treatment and medications as well as unaware of their symptoms. The mentally ill often have a limited support system. In contrast, populations of medical plans are more educated about medical conditions and services, like sonograms, cholesterol testing and CAT scans, and they are well versed in many medical procedures such as allergy shots, mammograms and colonoscopies, and so on. The symptoms of diabetes and heart disease, the correct medications for hyperglycemia and arthritis, and the appropriate procedures for a herniated disc or a broken ankle follow standard protocols even though these are ever changing and improving.

Isn't it interesting how most of us possess medical information without research? This thanks to the vast media around us. To access general medical care simply go to the doctor, clinic, lab or emergency room. For more complex procedures requiring a hospital stay call the number at the back of your health care card and get preauthorized for it. If a consumer is illiterate, no problem; most of the paperwork and calls to the managed care company are taken care of by others. Often the consumer pays a co-pay or deductible but rarely is a claim form needed. But behavioral health services start with often reluctant and even *combative* persons who may suffer with chronic illness and a medley of related problems. They may be incoherent upon arrival at a facility or over the phone. They may not have friends or next of kin to fill in the missing pieces of information about the patient's background. They may be in police custody. They may be suicidal or homicidal. They often suffer with untreated medical problems. Seriously mentally ill persons do not access services, they *get brought to services,* often by strangers. This makes a world of difference when processing an admission and accessing benefits.

Given the volume of conditions of dual origin, there have been attempts to coordinate managed behavioral care with managed medical care. According to some, the lack of coordination remains one of the industry's biggest failures (Moran, 2004).

In *The Need for Behavioral/Medical Integration and Opportunities for Psychology: A Perspective from Organized Healthcare,* Dr. Bruce L. Bobbitt (2007) discusses the need for integration between behavioral and medical healthcare and the MCO and MBHO because many major conditions such as cancer and heart disease may cause psychological conditions such as depression and anxiety. Psychologists, according to Dr. Bobbitt, have the desired training for this integrated approach. But, he admits that "one of the challenges to this integration is that patients prefer to talk with "professionals" and others who do not have doctoral degrees" (Bobbitt, 2005, p 15), or folks who do not have a lot of mysterious letters after their names such as PhD, Psych D, MA,LP,LCP, LPC.

A sad similarity between the MCO and the MBHO is the time waste, inefficiency, rising cost and declining quality of care that remains unaddressed by the industry in general. While it is still true that both our behavioral and medical care is the most advanced in the world due to progress in medical research and our free enterprise system, one would expect that an industry so refined over several decades would translate into higher costs. Documented nightmares are plentiful within all forms of managed care. One need only read *The Death of Compassion: The Endangered Doctor-Patient Relationship* by Jeffrey M.D. Thurston to get a sense of the ways in which managed care conflicts with the doctor's oath of "Do No Harm". The systemic problems at the managed care companies are the same.

As stated earlier, behavioral health care services are more complex than medical services because mental illnesses are less, well, "black and white" than medical illnesses. In fact, some still believe that mental health is not a *legitimate* field at all because of the vagueness of some of its science and the limited availability of quality outcome data. Perception is everything, so they say. The mentally ill still suffer from public bias. Cancer patients are called "heroes" while depressed patients are regarded skeptically by many. But make no mistake about it, mental health issues are equally painful and impacting on human life. Abnormalities of the brain and subsequent impaired life functioning require treatment as urgently as medical illnesses do. Further, the mentally ill often pose a grave danger to the rest of society and /or themselves. And finally, if Managed Behavioral Health and Managed Medical Health Care were one giant entity, think of the task of directing all these specialties under one managed care roof. Medical and mental health operations are already fiscally out of control, over centralized and impersonal.

There is little research about the separation of services though I have attempted to present its pros and cons. It would appear that any changes imposed on what we now have would hurt more than help. It may be time to save the concept but start from scratch. This author attempts to expose the nightmares in behavioral managed care to alert readers to the realities of this industry and how inefficient it is. The next case illustrates how a member can scam the system with bogus claims, how doctors can authorize hospital stays without legitimate cause, how a hospital can get away with providing poor services, and how the care manager can be tied up in bureaucracy while trying to manage a case.

Case in Point: 5/19/03 BCBS, Treatment Circus

Bill is a 54 year old male admitted to Timberstreet psychiatric hospital for depression, single episode, 296.23. Bill reportedly quit his job three days ago followed by an alleged suicide attempt with cocaine and Xanex, and continues to endorse suicide by gun. The precipitant reportedly was that he felt demeaned on his job and could not find a supervisor to report it to. Patient is divorced and lives with a roommate who refuses to take him back. He has been trying to contact friends who showed up to visit him but refuse to take him in while he looks for another job. Patient denies history of drug abuse. Patient reports if he is discharged to a shelter he will kill himself. Attending physician ordered Effexor 150, Remeron 45 and Lithium 300. Ritalin was then given to him over the weekend. The attending physician is seeking a county group home placement.

The care manager is very concerned that no UDA (urine drug analysis) has been performed to detect drugs in the patient's system, that a full drug history was not taken, that Ritalin(a very addictive drug) was given to a possible addict, and that the facility did not perform an adequate social assessment to determine patient's support system. (It is imperative that a patient have involvement with caring people whom the patient can turn to in case of a relapse). Worst of all, they did not ascertain this patient's risk of suicide. Does he own a gun? If so where is it? Has he had prior attempts? If so when and how? This is the "treating" facility's ethical responsibility!

This case was sent by the care manager to two doctors for review, each authorizing continued stay without any resolution to the care manager's concerns (which required beaucoup paperwork). Patient then discloses his history of drug use while at the facility, shows no signs of suicidality or symptoms of depression. So the original justification for the admission is gone. CM calls for a third doctor review in which the attending physician states that the patient will discharge–without a discharge plan! But when CM calls the next day to document the discharge plan (*more* paperwork and telephone calls) the facility reports that the patient remains there, prompting the CM to call for a FOURTH doctor review!! Following the completion of *umpteen* forms, documentation, telephone calls and hours later, the fourth doctor denies continued stay for this patient. Stay with me here...the attending physician then asks for an *appeal of the denial*! (which means *more* paperwork, staff involvement and another day in review). The appeal is lost, all parties agreeing with care manager that this patient needed to be in a shelter or group home with substance abuse treatment for his drug issues. After this paperwork catastrophe and shot nerves, patient finally left facility. But the managed care company ended up paying for a ten day stay for a patient who required a more thorough intake interview, a few days to stabilize and substance abuse treatment.

It should go without saying that micro management of procedures paired with poor quality services and unpredictable patients is not a winning combination for the American health care system.

Managing Alphabet Soup

It's confusing, it's shrouded, it's impersonal, it's perceptually negative, its' professionals and illnesses are in code. What is it? It's an MBHO! When the mental health professionals and the managed care industry with this whole other entity of health care coverage, **Managed Behavioral Health Care,** *is explained to people, they confess that they never heard of this (unless they have worked there).* As stated earlier by the author—if you never even heard of it, and had no idea it existed, and you cannot find it in the phone directory, the tendency is to be skeptical of it. If you have never seen an advertisement for *Magellan Behavioral Health* or other MBHOs then the perception of *"managed care"* and *"managed **behavioral** health care"* tends to be negative. There is no transparency and no public relations program to inform the public of what exactly goes on there..

Wallace Wilkins (2006) writes:

> "Managed Behavioral Health Care" is a positive, illusory spin for terminating, denying, preventing and interrupting health care to employees". He continues, "health care can only be managed when health care is delivered". (p 1)

My sentiments exactly!.

It is not surprising that many folks are confused about the mental health field in general. For instance, what is the difference among the following professionals: psychologists, psychiatrists, psychotherapists, social workers, and counselors? Over and over the author has heard parents report: "My son sees a counselor at school". Well, there is a big difference in the training of a school counselor and other counselors. In addition, some states use different labels for all these different professionals. The public cannot be blamed for their skepticism about the qualifications of "care managers" at the MBHO who ask a lot of personal questions and then make decisions about theirs or their loved one's mental health at some company they can't find in the phonebook! In this book the author will attempt to clear up many of the mysteries of Managed Behavioral Health Care. For starters, one way to explain your behavioral health care benefits and when you might access them would be to describe some situations:

Scenario #1

Let's say your husband has been drinking more than usual and coming home late from work and you know he's been feeling stressed from his job for a period of time. Tonight seems worse. He comes home, appears drunk, stalks into his room without saying hello, won't come out and tells you he's had it and he's going to kill himself. You call 911, the police come and coax him out but he is still threatening suicide. The police take him to the ER where he is assessed and it is determined that for his own safety he needs some psychiatric care in a psychiatric facility. A staff member asks you for your insurance card and calls the MBHO to find out which facility is in your network and what the limitations of the coverage are, and your husband is care flighted directly to a facility. When he arrives at the psychiatric facility, the admission and "stay" (time spent there) has to be "authorized". The facility calls your insurance company and the rest of the process will be explained in Part II.

Scenario #2

Or, let's take a less dramatic situation: your 10 year old comes home from school crying. You determine that she's been teased on the way home from school again today. Her grades have been dropping over the last several weeks and she is not sleeping well. You think she may benefit from talking to a therapist so you call your insurance company to find out what is covered, what is your co pay and to get a list of therapists in your area. You will reach the behavioral health care component (MBHO) of your health coverage. You'll tell them your situation, they will hook you up with a licensed professional who will get you the appropriate services.

Scenario #3

Here's a common situation: your next door neighbor suffers with schizophrenia. Most of the time, he appears normal to you but occasionally you've heard some screaming from his apartment or seen him wandering in the parking lot as if disoriented. One day you see an ambulance taking him off and he is gone for a few days. Your neighbor was probably taken to a psychiatric facility for "stabilization" or "medication evaluation or adjustment", etc. No doubt, the staff at the ER called his insurance carrier which led to an Intake Worker, which led to a Care Manager, very much like the author, and the process of admission and perhaps continued stay in that psychiatric facility was continued.

The events and issues described above may or may not involve persons with mental illnesses but these are clearly issues that require assessment by mental health professionals who are trained to gather a full family history, analyze symptoms that fit various pathologies, recommend protocol treatments, and rule out medical origins where needed.

The author's background as a mental health professional has included a journey through all sorts of providers of services from non- profit agencies and hospitals to private practices and public funded facilities, from therapists, "counselors", social workers and psychiatrists to licensed alcohol and drug counselors. The road I traveled included questionable practices, dubious pretend "patients", and practitioners who are more enabling than healing. "Pretend" patients are not real patients: they are criminals looking for a place to hide and a hot meal, or homeless folks looking for a few nights in a warm bed, or spouses kicked out of their homes or parents seeking to dump their unruly children. Due to the high volume of these pretend patients, some mental health professionals spend more time addressing social ills, rather than mental illnesses. While some mental health professionals enjoy this type of work, it is another drain on our system which raises the cost of behavioral health care. Don't misunderstand this author: there are many caring professionals who work with all sorts of human problems, but perhaps no other field allows for the existence of so many *pretenders*. Seriously mentally ill patients often go without services while our system is busy squandering its funds toward "pretend" patients. (More on "pretend patients" in a later section).

MANAGED CARE DICTIONARY OF TERMS

Policyholder	Consumer of health care, purchaser of policy, a.k.a. "member", once in treatment referred to as "patient".
Provider	One who provides services such as doctor, facility, treatment center, hospital, counselors, therapists, etc.
UR	Utilization Review, review of current status of a particular patient
UR	Utilization Reviewer, generic term for individual who conducts the review. This person may be from the Provider's side or the managed care side.
CM	Care Manager, individual Utilization Reviewer who works for managed care. Required Master's Level counselor or RN.
MNC	Medical Necessity Criteria. Criteria which determine authorization or denial of treatment
Denial	Denial of payment by managed care for a particular treatment for a particular individual Also referred to as "adverse determination", "non-authorization", "non-auth", "non-cert".
Authorization	Approval of payment of treatment by managed care. May be made by CM or managed care psychiatrist.

LOS

Length of Stay. How long an individual will be approved for a particular treatment.

LOC

Level of Care. Refers to severity of services, typically lowest LOC is outpatient therapy while hospitalization is highest LOC.

Appeal

Process by which a patient can contest a denial of payment of services for treatment.

Peer Review

Process by which a particular case may be reviewed by a managed care doctor and the provider doctor in the event the CM (care manager) is unwilling to approve continued treatment during a UR (utilization review). CM's are not authorized to deny treatment but a doctor may.

PART I   CHAP 3
THE PLAYERS & THE PROCESS

In a Deadbeat Corporation

The   players in the MBHO company, Corporate Officers, managers, supervisors, doctors, care managers, intake workers and support personnel attempt to accomplish their jobs despite the ever-present obstacles set up by regulatory agencies such as the State Department of Insurance, URAC, ERISA, HIPAA, JHACO, NCQA, licensing boards, and their very own internal process of Appeals.   In fact, these are just a handful of the regulations in place overwhelming the employees, the process of managing cases and serving policyholders.   Adding more regulations from the regulation happy government may seem preposterous but it continues to happen.   More about the reams of red tape in a later section.

The care manager (CM) is the very heart of the MBHO. It is the care manager who becomes intimately involved with the case, or, as intimate as one can be over the telephone! The CM takes in all the clinical information about the case, makes decisions about whether or not to authorize care and what level of care is appropriate for a particular patient.   It is the care manager who has overcome multiple obstacles to see the case through to its successful close. It is the care manager who applies the full agenda of quality patient care to each case. And indeed, it is the care manager's signature that will appear on that authorization, without which treatment cannot be assigned. But! The interference run by others in the managed care system prior to the time that authorization occurs is the nasty piece of the process that the reader will only see printed here. CMs come from many and varied licenses, education and training. More information about the job of the care manager (CM) will be discussed in a later section.

MBHOs are not at all the picture of a healthy, functional democracy that one would hope to see in a *BEHAVIORAL HEALTH CARE* setting...hello? Corporate types and their manager accessories put the squeeze on care managers until their signature authorizations are nothing more than robotic stamps. Doctors sometimes ride along independently, one of their main concerns protecting their risk level. Some of them are in the back pockets of some facilities, or blatantly working for these facilities, so the loopholes are certainly in place for unethical partnerships or conflicts of interest. And sometimes, like care managers, doctors may be intimidated and opt to toe the corporate line. The managers and supervisors are chosen for their knowledge of the policies and regulations and a "corporate" personality. But there's something sleazy about these folks; superficial personality traits and an empty soul seem to characterize most of them that I have worked for. Oh, they may have started out umpteen years ago with good intentions when managed care was just an ideal.   Then, to survive in this business today, personality and ability to maneuver and manipulate and crunch numbers became more important than compassion for patients.

THE PLAYERS: *"Chain, Chain, Chain, Chain of Fools"*
Corporate

Corporate is interested in profits.   For obvious reasons this group is not focused on quality of care for patients, except where they are forced to be by regulation.   They're not philanthropists, they don't take an oath to "do no harm", they don't enter this line of work out of some sense of altruism. They're business people. This author is well aware that good upstanding business people are to be found everywhere.   But managed care companies are in this to make a profit.   The author has no criticism with this; we live in a capitalist society which has served us well.   But this group tends to be *less knowledgeable* of the mental health field than is needed to wield the kind of decision making power that they have within it. For a peek at the power these individuals hold, see the letter from Keith Dixon, CEO of Cigna in Part II Chap 1.

Supervisors/Floor Managers

Think "drill Sergeant", enforcer, even "bully" and you will have somewhat of a image of the supervisors of care managers. They are not necessarily intelligent nor upstanding, but they possess the power to intimidate and play mind games on their underlings, the care managers. Every team of care managers has a supervisor who more or less keeps everyone in line with what I call the mentality of "scarcity"; approval is scarce, providers are scarce and opinions from care managers should be scarce as well. This describes the Aetna plan. Managers want to maintain power and influence so they also play politics with providers while undermining care managers. This goes something like this: "Mr./Ms Provider, I will provide you with many patients if you create more of the services we need to protect our bottom line". This describes Blue Cross Blue Shield. And, last but hardly least, managers want to swamp care managers with administrative busy work and mind numbing computer data entry so that they are too worn out to have any input at all. This describes Cigna.

Upper Management/Mid-Management

Then there's Management who oversees supervisors and a medley of levels in between. Upper Management folks attend meetings, conduct other meetings and intimidate supervisors to lean on care managers. They make policies, consult attorneys, develop public relations and training programs, and oversee the center. They include the Chief Medical Director, VP and President. Some are trained experienced mental health professionals but all spew the corporate mantras and dabble in politics. What are the chances of a care manager rising to this level? It appears that some Fool's Handbook determined that the main characteristic for "rising" from care manager to supervisor and then to manager is the ability to smile a lot, steel nerves with a heart of stone, and a "flexible nature", (can speak from both sides of the mouth).

Psychiatrists

Psychiatrists are medical doctors who attend additional years of training in brain functioning; they can and do prescribe medications and conduct therapy if they choose. The psychiatrist is a *medical doctor first* with additional training in mental and psychological conditions and brain functioning.

The doctors of the MBHOs started out as big players in the decision making. For almost two decades it was believed that the doctors should be making more of the decisions today. After all, doctors insure credibility, bring research based, quality protocols and results based practices to the mental health treatment. Best of all, they are also interested in patient care, having taken the Hippocratic Oath. But doctors have become somewhat marginalized in the managed care industry today. Job retention requires that they please the people above them who are often not well-meaning. They are treated with slightly more deference than the care manager, who also went to school for years and years and has miles of experience with mental illnesses. At the same time MBHOs are structured in such a way as to leave doctors with more "wiggle room" (opportunities for corruption). A Psychiatrist for an MBHO may also have a private practice and be a provider with the same managed care company. A doctor may even be the medical director of a facility that is also a provider of the same managed care company. Does this sound kosher to you? It happens.

Psychologists

Some healthcare organizations have one or more psychologists whose main usefulness is to recommend various types of psychological tests for members, particularly when the care manager cannot diagnose a member, or where the member's complaint is not clear. Their function is pretty specific and their training includes medical areas as well as psychological area.

In the absence of the staff psychologist, a care manager in need of advice and/or information would consult the staff psychiatrist instead. How are psychologists and psychiatrists different? The former is a Ph.D. level mental health professional with training and internship experience in medicines, counseling and testing methods and interpretation. The psychiatrist is a medical doctor first who after completing medical school takes additional training in mental and behavioral abnormalities and treatments for them.

Claims

The valiant servants in Claims work tirelessly to come up with a believable bill to send to you, the policyholder, after all the games are played among your dubious "friends", the insurance company, the managed care company and the providers. Not that any of the paperwork is coordinated; that makes too much sense! If the policyholder accepts the bill as believable, it will probably get paid to the provider without too much question or resistance. As you can imagine, the fireworks start when the bill you receive does not meet your *math* standards. Many managed care mishaps can be attributed to their Claims Department. Fines are given when claims are not paid on time. Claims complaints and delays are another sad outcome of poor management and bureaucracy.

Care Managers

Once the MBHO has brief information about the case from the Intake Specialist, there is a significant amount of additional very personal information that needs to be obtained. This is the first goal of the care managers. As stated earlier, these are the professionals who get assigned to the case, "work the case", review and document the case and complete the authorizations on the case. Care managers monitor the treatment of a patient with the provider by telephone. Care managers initiate a doctor review when needed, and follow up on the results. Care managers design discharge plans and follow the case via telephone once treatment is complete. One could say these folks know the case and the patient more intimately than the rest of the managed behavioral health care personnel. Though the relationship between the care manager and policyholder is not a face to face one these "tele-counselors can be considered consultants. They don't actually counsel patients, they *make decisions for* patients based on their knowledge and training in mental health. Since not all providers deliver care in the most updated and meticulous way that they should, care managers provide some oversight while the patient is in treatment.

Care Management: An Admirable Art

As stated in the introduction to this section, care managers come from many parts of the mental health field. *School*

Counselors have training in working with children and adolescents in a school environment on a short term or crisis basis. *Social Workers* are trained in community services and general situations such as career search, child abuse and legal issues. *Licensed Professional Counselors* are trained in mental illnesses and substance abuse care and treatment as well as counseling techniques. Still, all care managers can be called the "front line" of the managed care company.

Care managers are Master's Level graduates, some with doctoral status, and require licensing by the State. Each one of these professionals is required to complete an internship in actual face to face intervention with patients. An additional six years of experience in face to face counseling is required after licensing by the state is obtained. Each license requires ethical treatment of clients for the renewal of the license. Care managers in managed care companies risk their licenses every day! The author hopes to establish for readers an appreciation for the skills, experience and training which can elevate the CM to consultant status. But as far as the general public knows, they may be "some insurance workers", or "some (generic type) counselors" or worse, some "corporate-type persons". But CMs must be first *specialists* in mental health, not business or insurance. No other field requires of their professionals that they possess knowledge from other fields as does the MBHO.

CMs are mental health providers, company representatives, coordinators with medical care, knowledgeable about certain plans and the insurance business and, oh yes, computer technicians and data entry clerks! More will be said later about the care manager's heavy load of data entry. But trust me, there is little aid for a care manager juggling time limits and an overwhelming case load with help for computer problems (at least, not in a timely manner). Often, there's a form to complete for computer assistance...

Since the field of mental health and its varying professionals is so broad most graduates of mental health programs move around sampling every area of service before entering managed care.   Few graduates have designs on becoming a care manager at a managed care company at the early stages of their careers.   As a result, the typical care manager brings much more to the job then the minimum requirements described previously. Chances are the care manager even has a prior career of experiences to tap into. The author is a example of this: I was trained and educated in counseling following twenty two years in the field of Education, as a teacher, administrator, teacher trainer and college professor.

Additionally, the typical care manager comes to this position with years of experience with every imaginable population from mentally ill to socially challenged– birth to elderly. Nurse care managers bring an additional knowledge of medical issues as they relate to the social/emotional and mental conditions of patients. If one is unfamiliar with medical issues, one is expected to become familiar with them. Though they are inadequately trained by the MBHO about insurance policies, case management and computer programs, they are expected to "fly from the seat of their pants" so to speak. Ongoing training was available in the MBHOs that I worked in but it was never adequate.

When acquaintances become aware of the background and training of a licensed counselor out come the questions that people struggle with on a daily basis -- about medications, their elderly parents with memory impairments, their children with attention deficit problems, their personal experiences with depression or anxiety, and their marital problems! Obviously some number of the population appreciates the expertise of the trained mental health professional. Not true among the management folks at the MBHOs.

The Lowly Care Manager

Despite the fact that care managers are the most familiar with the case, their autonomy has slowly eroded and in some managed care companies, they are merely names on an authorization—puppets for corporate and managers. They are often strangled with over regulation and they are being squeezed by the greedy hands of Corporate. Many times they are abused with unrealistic evaluation procedures, timing devices and schedules. They are asked to do many tasks outside of their area of specialty with little or no support. In recent years, care managers have been intimidated to change their decisions to suit corporate agendas. They are threatened with poor performance assessments and consequential loss of raises or promotions. I know of cases where care managers have been unjustly fired on bogus charges of "poor performance" due to their authorization decisions. I have witnessed supervisors who ordered care managers to authorize care where criteria for care was not met and to send cases to peer review when criteria was met. It's equal opportunity corruption. There are doctors who will do the bidding of the corporation and deliver up denials or approvals as needed. There are Intake Specialists to get to know so that care managers can receive clear and thorough information about each case. There are supervisors ready with the whip at the care manager's back.

Policyholders are often quick to blame the CM and less willing to recognize the part that the providers play in damaged care. A common complaint among policyholders to the care manager is: "Who are you to be making decisions about length of stay for my son, my mother, etc...." Be aware that the facility reviewers are, 1. not held to the same standards as care managers at the MBHO, and, 2. are often under severe constraints in giving quality updated clinical information to care managers at the MBHO. They are subjected to missing charts that they must then chase down or compete for with doctors. They must peel through horrendous handwriting samples for which doctors are notorious. The charts they read from are haphazardly organized for various personnel to use, and tend to be least of all set up for utilization reviewers to access or use. The public needs to know this. Face facts: they are willing to sell a service through pressure from *their supervisors*. Conflicts of interests permeate all of damaged care!

In light of what the reader has been told about the credentials of care managers, perhaps less skepticism and negativity will be expressed toward these professionals. Likewise, when policyholders become aware that it is in the hospital's best interest (in profits) to extend the stay of a patient and even exaggerate the patient's condition, more policyholders will question the providers as much as the MBHO care managers.

On a lighter note, just hang around an experienced CM's desk long enough and witness a cross between the shows "Let's Make a Deal" and "Survivor". There are providers who are "in network" and those who are "out of network" . Surprise, surprise, these lists are usually not up to date leaving the Intake Specialists (described in the next section), CMs and Claims folks to scramble for the correct identity and cost of a particular service. One can view this scramble on any given day. There are benefits for inpatient care but only for five days after which you may as well ransom your home and kids. There are hospital regulations for inpatient stays and managed care guidelines for who is eligible for admission. These often don't match up and are pretty useless. There are charts, cheat sheets, manuals and diagrams. There are ever changing codes for every imaginable treatment and diagnosis. I knew a CM who was a genius with multi tasking: she could commiserate with the patient on line one, and conference in the provider while arguing with the insurance company on line two– all while inputting the entire fiasco onto the computer! Oh, and it is always *urgent!* No matter what the issue is, it's crisis work and very stressful. CMs are the un-mined diamonds of the managed behavioral healthcare industry.

Intake Specialists

I call these brave folks "Face the Nation" warriors. These individuals risk their very lives to pick up the violently ringing telephones at the madhouse that is the Managed Care Organization. They do not know who will be on the other end, what they will want or say, what language they will be speaking, if they will even have the correct number. Still they answer, over and over. They are timed, they are taped and weary as they sit in their cubes enduring a great deal of stress. MBHOs monitor how often the phones are picked up and how long the calls are. They keep close tabs on the so called "abandonment rate" (when the policyholder hangs up prior to the connection). Intake workers must be courteous and have good computer skills plus have knowledge of mental health issues, managed care, behavioral health care policies, and benefits. Of course they must know everyone in the office and what they do so they know how to route the call. They must be able to build the case, open the case, prep the case, clean up the case, document what they did with the case, and transfer the case. They are underpaid and job turnover is high.

Support Personnel

Bachelor's level staff handle follow up calls to patients, sending out packets of information, entering non confidential data. There are never enough of these folks.

Appeals Department

This department handles cases where treatment has been denied payment. Policyholders can appeal any decision they do not agree with. The most qualified folks to re-examine the files are care managers and doctors. Surprisingly, there are real "overturns" (reversal of denial decisions) through this process. More policyholders need to know about this vehicle in advance of accessing any benefits and make more frequent use of it. Although a letter is sent with information about Appeals at the time of a denial, this is usually a tumultuous time for the policyholder who usually is a patient receiving care. There are time limits on reviewing and rendering decisions in Appeal cases. If an appeal fails to get the policyholder the desired outcome, he or she can request an Independent Review (IRO).

Joe & Joan Q Public

Call them Policyholders/Members/Clients/Patients. These are the folks supposedly served by the MBHO. Management and doctors at the MBHO in general *do not have contact with the policyholders*, but Intake and CMs have telephone contact, while Claims has mail or telephone contact. Supervisors sometimes handle irate customers and those policyholders threatening to sue. It bears repeating: *None of the contact mentioned is face to face.* In fact, the reader will not be able to even LOCATE his or her managed care company. No one actually goes to the managed care company except managed care personnel: it's all part of the very impersonal and protected shield in which they operate. The giant pot of soup sours...

Insurance Companies and Managed Care

Readers are familiar with some of the bigger names such as Aetna, Blue Cross Blue Shield, Humana, United Health Care, Cigna, Prudential, Optum, etc. These are the insurance companies and managed care companies which offer mental health insurance via a policy. These policies spell out conditions and *approved services* or *benefits* to large and small groups of employees such as those working at AT&T and TI and Bell Helicopter as well as Mom & Pop businesses and even individual citizens. That's you, the taxpayer, you, the policyholder, you, sometimes the "patients" calling for help and others who never requested help and end up in the ER. The insurance companies have expectations for how they want their benefits "spent", as do the employers that purchase their policies for their employees. There is continuous conflict between these business partners both competing for the same level of care at the cheapest price.

Providers

The providers, also referred to as "services" or "service providers", render the needed mental health care. They are the many hospitals, clinics, doctors and therapists, treatment centers, halfway houses and psychiatric facilities who consider themselves business partners with the MBHO as well. Therein lies the dubious relationship that poses harm to policyholders and taxpayers. While the policyholder and their employers seek the very best (often most expensive care), the insurance company is looking for the least expensive quality care that falls within their benefit guidelines. Providers are looking for volume, profit and maintenance of their reputations. And the managed care company is, well, manipulating all these entities so all will spend the benefits wisely, AND make a profit! If you haven't guessed it by now, there are ever changing rules, guidelines and definitions everywhere. Contracts are constantly nuanced and updated. There's legalese, fine print and risk for all involved; some even conflict with each other!

THE PROCESS: *"Got coverage?"*
Alphabet Soup Spells ...

As stated earlier, the mental health field is riddled with titled professionals and their licenses, such as Social Workers (LMSWs), Licensed Professional Counselors (LPCs), Nurses (MSRNs), and Drug and Alcohol Counselors (LCDC–depending upon licensing State). Likewise, Managed Care offers many different types of plans. Readers recognize these plans as **the alphabet:** HMO, PPO, POS and MBHO. Further, MBHOs, already a "carve out" from MCOs, can contract out *their* services to a SAMHSA or to an ASO! Some employers also opt for an EAP (Employee Assistance Program) instead of a MBHO carve out. Whichever way they go, we have "capitation" going on with the providers of the services! This gobbledegook does not help the policyholder in a time of crisis! (Carve outs and capitation discussed in other section).

It's all very confusing and may even be deliberately so. Can consumers complain in an environment of chaos that they have no control over at a time in their lives when they are in crisis or at least in need? In the end, consumers may end up with an excess of bills and other associated paperwork from several different companies that are usually not well coordinated working on his or her "case". One notice tells you that your bill was covered per your plan, and the next notice tells you there is some remaining amount you need to pay. None of these notices are clear, even with this little *glossary* of sorts in the back for you to interpret the codes! These generally contain lots of managed care terminology and don't help much after the shock of the bill itself. Often the consumer doesn't even recognize the names of the companies on these bills. The recipients of all this paper are probably thinking; "I paid that–didn't I?" This *secret language,* or "professional terminology" as they would describe it, is nothing more than condescending to the policyholders and perhaps even deliberately obscure.

Once again I am compelled to assert that *"Too many cooks spoil the brew"* and that *brew* is beginning to foam at this point!

Step 1 Intake

Today, accessing mental health benefits can be daunting under a managed care plan. (Mental Health, A Report of the Surgeon General, 17, p 8). Sure, more of us have "access", but to what? As was stated earlier, the function of managed care is to connect you, the policyholder, with services such as therapists, psychiatrist and treatment centers within the guidelines of your specific benefits and your particular condition. Hopefully your call will not fall into *"The Queue"* –the big black hole of waiting on hold to the tunes of the MBHO medley of musical selections. If you *do* get through successfully, you will reach "Intake", where your basic questions are answered like: "Am I insured and what does my policy cover vs. what do I need?"

Then there is the issue of "in-network" vs. "out of network" providers, which is based on contracts between managed care and providers who will settle for pittance pay-outs. You are skeptical about seeing a "mental health provider" in the first place, now you learn that some are "in" and some are "out". The Intake specialist also answers these questions. For example, you had hoped to see a therapist who was recommended by your cousin only to learn that the therapist is "not in network" and you have no "out of network benefits". What does this mean exactly? Bluntly put, if you want to see your cousin's therapist you will have to pay for it yourself. As a personal note, the author went to an "in network" hospital following an accident but was treated by several doctors, one of whom was "out of network". Needless to say, consumers beware! Make sure to ask anyone who even briefly touches you in a hospital if he/she is covered by your plan. What? You are unconscious or too ill to check this out? Sorry, here's your bill. Location is another big bugaboo. If you live, for example, in a "geo-remote" area, some plans allow you to see an out of network provider, while some expect you to drive to Canada for the nearest in network doctor—even for surgery!

Policyholders become even angrier when they learn that there are more restrictions placed upon their access to services. Like when you attempt to enter a hospital for psychiatric care and are denied services because "you don't meet *medical necessity criteria* for inpatient care". This can be especially frustrating for the policyholder who tends to believe that after paying premiums, this type of service should be rendered automatically because it is seems necessary to the policyholder. So all these matters have to be hammered out before the policyholder gets connected with services, or gets transferred to someone else for even more questioning.

By this time, the policyholder is very relaxed—NOT!

Next, it would seem that they would have to get to know you very well to find out exactly what you need. Here, the author emphasizes VERY well–as in all your personal goings on, deepest feelings and most darkest secrets. The Intake Person you first spoke to is not qualified to do that piece; only a licensed clinician is. Enter the care manager.

Step 2 Intake Care Manager

The strengths and skills of the CM have been discussed in a previous section. The Intake care manager is the specific CM who will telephonically interview the policyholder to ascertain if admission to a psychiatric facility is needed. The questions are very personal and for some callers very intrusive. If the care manager has to use a *template* created by the company, the questions often sound irrelevant and even stupid!   The questions may be in "managed care speak" such as "Are you at risk of harm to yourself or others?" Why, this is not even correct English! Don't these two types of "harm" deserve separate questions?! The skilled Intake CM works up gently to these personal questions, asking first to confirm name, address, policy number, etc. When care managers are allowed to use their own words, they step up to the plate with their interviewing and listening skills, their compassion and empathy for the caller and this will be evident to the caller. The CM will take a detailed history and record your current medications, symptoms and experience with treatment. Next, the CM will attempt to make a preliminary diagnosis of your problem.

What is the nature of your problem? A diagnosis is an illness or condition substantiated by the mental health professionals' Bible, the DSM. The DSM (Diagnostic Statistical Manual), defines in specific terms each mental condition known to current researchers. Mental illnesses such as Depression or Bipolar Disorder have identifiable symptoms and presentations to support their diagnoses. They are not pulled out of thin air as some might believe!

But what if your problem does not appear in this so-called Bible? Poppycock! Every condition known to man or woman is in the DSM. And if it is not, it will be in the revised next edition of the DSM. The DSM is like "Prego" tomato sauce. Remember, "It's in there!"? Pedophilia? It's in there!; Kleptomania? It's in there! Oppositional Defiant Disorder? In the DSM; Chronic Alcoholism? It's in there! ; Caffeine Withdrawal? In the DSM; Selective Mutism? It's in there!; Pain Disorder? It's in there! If you don't think you have something, there may be a diagnosis for that too.

The problem is never that your illness is *not* in the DSM; the problem is that your policy does not **cover** everything in the DSM. Now, most people are not very happy to hear that their policy has no benefits for what ails them. Face the Nation will inform you of this early on in the phone call and take your expletive remarks also prior to your conversation with an Intake Care Manager; hopefully by then you will have come up with a *covered* illness to have!

At some point when the CM is comfortable with the information, he or she may evaluate your needs for "level of care". Level of care (LOS) describes the intensity and frequency of the treatment the patient/policyholder requires. If a patient is suicidal and has the means to harm him/herself, the CM will recommend hospitalization, the highest level of care. The next lowest level of care may be "partial hospitalization" or "day hospital". The next lowest level of care would be "Intensive Outpatient Treatment". This service is available in a hospital or clinic; the patient attends two to five days per week for a limited period of time depending upon the severity of the patient's condition. The CM assigns this level of care when a patient needs a great deal of structure and support but is not suicidal. Many substance abuse providers and treatments for adolescents offer partial or full day programs in which the patients go home in the evenings. The next lowest level of care is *outpatient counseling.* The patient is assigned to a counselor/social worker/therapist who specializes in the patient's complaint in a location closest to the patient. Patient goes to scheduled appointments for a length of time determined by the care manager and provider. Six visits may be authorized at first. In six weeks, the Out Patient CM reviews the case to determine if more visits are necessary. A co-pay is collected from the policyholder and the provider may or may not file a claim form. Unfortunately, the change of hands from the Intake CM to the Out Patient CM is not always smooth. This is to be expected in a large bureaucracy.

Review is a very serious and complex process in the patient's treatment. Some policyholders do not know exactly what a review is and they assume it is another arbitrary decision about whether or not to continue to pay for treatment. Although much depends upon the parameters of the managed care company and the patient's policy, the conscientious CM (those who have not yet been fired) attempts to learn about the patient's response to treatment, the current outcome of the treatment, the patient's acknowledgment of improvement, etc. to determine if extended treatment is warranted. This is tricky because the patient is not directly consulted; the service provider is the one who supplies this information. The message that the CM wants to hear is that the patient has made significant progress and there is a "discharge plan" in place.

(This is what the patient plans to do after treatment is over in terms of maintaining improvements).

In some instances (which will be described shortly), the care manager will get all the necessary information about the policyholder second hand from the psychiatric facility or hospital. This is protocol when the policyholder attempts suicide, or threatens to hurt someone else, or is behaving bizarrely, and is rushed by ambulance to one of these facilities. Another situation involves police escorted patients brought to a hospital for admission. Either the court has ordered this or police determine that the patient is dangerous to him/herself or others. In these cases, the patient is incoherent or even uncooperative and the CM will have to obtain information about him or her from the nurse in charge, the admitting doctor or another care manager called a UR (Utilization Reviewer). These other care managers do the same job but work for "the other side", as we used to say. They are viewed by managed care as adversaries most of the time who view the CM at the MBHO as the purse string holders ready to deny coverage. However, these opposite side CMs should work as partners toward the patient's success in treatment. While this is the ideal, this is not always the case and the providers become one more source of stress always challenging professional opinions and recommendations, always seeking more care where less may be indicated.

One could say that the MBHO care manager is not only a kind of shock absorber at the beginning of a case, but also the link between the policyholder and the managed care company and between the service provider and the patient. The job is precarious, nerve wracking, ambiguous, stressful and for some, a "rush". In short, without the care manager the managed care company could not proceed with its business goals. (The care manager's job has also been described in Part I Chap 3 under Player's).

Step 4 Provider/Services

Go here, get better. Maybe. Maybe temporarily, then relapse and return to Step 1. Somehow, the providers are not viewed as skeptically as the managed care company or insurance company. But it should be noted that there are substandard hospitals and facilities out there. And there are unscrupulous and money hungry doctors and therapists out there. Sad to say, some are selfishly motivated to give treatment that is unwarranted or to keep a patient longer than is necessary for their own bottom line. In the original managed care concept, these tendencies were to be reined in. While these "ulterior motives" are infrequent among providers, managed care still needs to be reined in!

Step 5 Claims   "Don't call us, we'll call YOU"

Skip this step if you get your bills, pay up, paid the co-pays to the doctor, hospital, therapist, anesthesiologist, lab, and so on. But if the bills are wrong, call Claims; wait forever. Don't pay up? Claims will call you.

Step 6 Appeals

Skip this step if you agree with everything the managed care company has done on your behalf while you were receiving treatment. Don't like the decisions or how you were treated? Call this number and get ready to fight, or "appeal" your case. Another doctor will review the information and may *uphold* (agree with the original denial) or *overturn* (change the denial to an approval) the original decision. If the second decision is not what you expected, another level of appeal called an IRO (Independent Review Organization) is available in some plans. Few people know that one can also threaten to inform the State Insurance Board for an unacceptable decision.

The reader is reminded again that the following players are not actually personally involved with the policyholder during the above process unless something unusual occurs: the CEO,

Medical Director, Doctors, Management, Supervisors, Public Relations, Human (ha!) Relations, President and Vice President of the company. Yet all of these have more power (and higher salaries) than the lowly care manager.

One way to explain the process in a more concrete way is to illustrate some common cases. The following are some examples of cases that come into the MBHO phone line and how they are handled.

Scenario #1

Let's say your mother is feeling depressed and you had hoped to get her into a psychiatric facility for treatment. You skip the call to the managed care company and bring her to such a facility and have her assessed by one of their staff and present your insurance card. The staff calls the managed care company to give the results of the assessment (we call this the *clinical information*) and informs you that your mother "does not meet the medical necessity criteria for inpatient care" and has therefore been denied payment for the treatment. Though the staff and perhaps even the admitting psychiatrist may recommend that your mother be admitted for treatment, your insurance company is not willing to cover the cost. The psychiatric facility is VERY interested in admitting your mother. The managed care company refuses to cover it. Naturally the managed care company appears to be the culprit. Or, if your mother does meet the medical necessity criteria spelled out by the managed care company she may be admitted for treatment with an initial stay of only three days.

Intro to Medical Necessity Criteria

The MBHO's criteria for admission to a psychiatric facility is based on "medical necessity criteria". MNC or medical necessity criteria for hospital admission usually means that without treatment, the patient may hurt him/herself or others. If care is denied and a serious incident of harm occurs, both hospital and managed care companies are liable. Were it not for this *risk* factor, there would still be the *cost* factor. Beds and staff, including doctors, are limited and costly. Many mental illnesses can be treated at a *lower level of care*, for example with the correct medication or access to an immediate crisis therapist, etc.

From a care manager's perspective, hospitalization is a traumatic experience-a little known fact–particularly for children and the elderly. It is invasive, geared only to crisis stabilization and the "inmates" are frightening, yet the patient will be assessed for whether they interact with others or isolate themselves. The rules are strict, one may not leave when one feels like it and it remains on one's record forever. So it is a last resort reserved for those who need to be kept safe because they are in a state of crisis, those who are in imminent danger of harm to themselves or others, or those so psychotic that their functioning is impaired, or those unable to care for their daily basic needs such as eating and bathing.

Still, the author has encountered calls from policyholders who view psychiatric facilities as retreats for "processing" their "issues", or placements for their unruly teenagers, or refuge after an especially difficult divorce, or a respite for the battered spouse, a bed for the homeless, a hideout for a parolee... the list goes on.   Do you believe the facilities want to weed out these scavengers? Not so much if the facility is unethical and more interested in profits.   As far as these facilities are concerned, all are welcomed as long as the straggler has an insurance card. Some unethical facilities will hire some equally unethical UR (utilization reviewer) staff who will portray the policyholder as truly ill, citing the patient as "suicidal with a plan" and having "poor sleep, poor appetite, poor concentration", and whatever it takes to convince the MBHO to approve treatment. With the embellished clinical, the patient gets admitted and the insurance company pays the bill. End of story. (The author also worked for one such facility prior to being a care manager) But when a well-trained experienced care manager is on the case, probing questions and careful analysis of the symptoms shed more light on the identity and actual needs of the patient. And, yes, this may result in a denial of the requested care. Has this author seen the "denial" button pushed too often by care managers? You bet: there are abuses going on both ways. To compound the MNC issue, it can be easily misinterpreted, and different for different plans and facilities. (MNC discussed again in Part III)

Scenario #2

In this case, the policyholder is coherent and functional and also requests help for a family member. This time, the instructions on the back of the insurance card are followed and a call is placed to the MBHO. Face the Nation picks up the phone on "Q". (More about the Queue in the next section) The caller describes the situation and requests outpatient treatment such as a therapist or a psychiatrist because the caller or caller's husband or child has a problem. The Intake specialist may take some basic information before transferring the caller to an Outpatient CM who will ask some questions then give some referrals. Typically, these referrals are to counselors and psychiatrists located within 25 miles of the patient's residence.

Scenario #3

Or, you are in a crisis, yet functional enough to call the number on the back of your insurance card to find out what to do. You are unable to sleep, your thoughts are racing, you feel frightened, your heart is pounding, you've been off your prescribed meds for two weeks and you live alone.... The Intake Specialist will ask you if you are feeling suicidal to assess the degree of severity of your crisis. You are too foggy to answer, or you think: " maybe yes..." You are quickly transferred to a triage/crisis CM, also known as an Intake CM. This is likely to result in a recommendation and authorization for an admission to a psychiatric facility. You will be instructed to go to the facility and be assessed again by their staff before being admitted, or an ambulance may be called for you. This is clear cut and a less common scenario.

Scenario #4

Now, let's say that you, the policyholder, just wonder if treatment is needed or want to learn about all the treatment options available. After calling the number on the back of the insurance card, you would ask for information and be transferred to a triage/crisis care manager. The CM will look up your policy to see your benefits and ask about the person needing services, and the problems and symptoms. Remember that this is a highly trained professional who does not take your call lightly and who is skilled at assessing as well as treating many different populations with many types of mental and emotional disorders. This individual is a Licensed Professional Counselor or a Licensed Masters Social Worker or a Master's Level Nurse. If the care manager assesses your situation and recommends that you go to an outpatient therapist, a list of "in network" providers will be given for the caller to call and schedule an appointment.

Scenario #5 *The road less traveled...*

QUICK! YOU'RE IN A CRISIS! WHO YA GONNA CALL?

a. The police, b. An ambulance, c. 911, d. Your friendly managed care company. If you answered "d" you are unusual for sure, but to the managed care company this is the *correct* answer. For the rest of us who *did not* call the managed care company, the process goes something like this: The policyholder goes directly to the service needed either voluntarily with mother or spouse or friend, or involuntarily (escorted by police and ambulance). In these cases it is difficult to know whether or not the hospital stay will be authorized by the managed care company. It will be up to the hospital provider to make that call and plead for approval on behalf of the patient.

Hospitalized policyholders are extremely vulnerable particularly if they do not have a relative, friend or guardian who can contribute to the admission process with medical and mental history information about the patient. Intake workers take thousands of calls throughout the day, many from facility UR (Utilization Reviewers) and nurses who work for the hospitals. These calls will next go to the Inpatient Care Managers working at the MBHO. These are the care managers who get the case *after the patient has been admitted*_into the hospital or psychiatric facility. Usually, one to three days have already been authorized at the time of intake through the contract with that hospital. This is re-negotiated regularly through reviews, so the care manager will have to know what has been agreed to. The Inpatient CM is responsible for periodic *review* of the case to assess the quality of the patient's care, to determine if more time is needed for care, and to help facilitate the discharge planning. The CM wants to know: What is being done with the patient? What medicines will the patient receive? How much longer will the treatment take?, and, What is the follow up plan after discharge? As stated earlier, care managers become somewhat more intimately involved with a patient and develops more personal responsibility on this type of case even though there is no face to face contact. Unfortunately, the definition of a hospital stay under managed care is a brief time of 5-7 days or even 3-5 days, unless a case is very serious.

Patient Dumping

This is not my terminology folks; it is a recognized though dubious practice among private psychiatric facilities and public hospitals. Talk about the vulnerability of a patient who admits to a hospital- this takes the soup AND the cake! If a patient does not have enough insurance covering hospitalization for his/her current condition, the private facility (usually psychiatric facilities) will keep a patient long enough to collect fees under an "emergency" admission provision available through public assistance, perhaps 3-5 days. When the benefits are exhausted, the patient gets transferred to a public facility. For patients with no coverage, the "dumping" will happen much sooner. This results is interruption of care, debt to the public facility, (which by law must treat them), and you and I paying $35 for an aspirin the next time we admit to a hospital!

Peer Review Process

When the care manager and the care manager (UR) on the provider side are unable to agree on the member's treatment for whatever reason, the care manager has one really useful tool. A MBHO psychiatrist is either consulted with or will conduct what is called a **Peer Review** or *Doctor to Doctor*

Review, or *"PA".* For a short period of time the case is out of the care manager's hands and two doctors will decide upon the destiny of the member. The MBHO doctor will telephonically review the case with the doctor who is directly treating the patient (also called "treatment provider" or "treatment doctor"). As stated in an earlier section, the relationship between the MBHO and their "network" of providers is symbiotic and contractual. In contrast, the CM (care manager) and UR(care manager at the facility) are in an adversarial relationship: the MBHO CM leans toward *less* treatment and the provider UR leans toward *more* treatment. The managed care doctor must render an impartial decision as to whether the patient will continue with treatment ("continued stay") or the patient will have to discharge from the facility (denial) and in some cases, if the admission should have been made in the first place. By issuing too many approvals the doctor gains a less than positive reputation within the MBHO (similar to the way care managers are treated). In the meantime, the CM is bound by multiple regulations to get the information to the doctor ahead of time, gain a time on his schedule, play phone tag with the provider's office, get a decision within 24 hours, notify all parties telephonically, send out written notifications and document and all this *accurately* to boot! CMs usually send cases for Peer Review when they see reason to deny continued stay but lack the authority to do so. Those care managers who pursue this avenue often are regarded highly by the MBHO managers, yet the process of arranging the Peer Review is archaic and tedious to say the least. Go figure! If on the other hand the health plan is a PPO, which is "non-risk" plan like BCBS, then the care manager is viewed not so highly because managed care collects a flat fee for serving these patients: nothing is gained by denying these patients care, but everything is gained in public relations if they are approved for care. This treatment of CMs was sorely felt by this author when I managed Aetna and then moved to BCBS. After a case gets a formal denial from a doctor to doctor review, the patient-policyholder can contest the denial through an appeals process. Another bureaucratic process plagued by multitudinous regulations and exasperating protocols, appeals may result in an "overturn" (denial becomes an approval) or an "uphold" (denial remains) after review by another doctor. It's what I like to call Decision Recycling, and everyone knows they can manipulate this process as well. If a care manager sends a case to Peer Review and it is returned as a denial, that confirms that the CM has good instincts about a case. In addition, If the denial is *appealed* by the policyholder and the appeal is returned as an *uphold (denial remains)*, that also confirms that the CM is on the ball.

PART I CHAP 4

JOURNEY INTO MBHO

To Hell and Back

In *We-make-our-own-laws Texas*, I have worked for two Managed Behavioral Health Care organizations which together manage many well known insurance carriers, one more strangulated in bureaucracy, over regulation and questionable practices than the other. Three of these are Cigna, Aetna and Blue Cross Blue Shield. Though they are staffed with highly educated and trained professionals, these employees are squeezed out of the decision-making process in favor of the corporate folks in charge of the managed care purse strings. These are the CEOs and their accessories, the supervisors and mid managers.

Who pays for this mismanagement?   Taxpayers, policyholders, business owners, employees, employers alike pay with increased premiums and higher taxes, all in an effort to "hold down the cost of health care"!! In terms of quality we all pay again. Bureaucracy and unplugged loopholes translates into wasted time, wasted money and fewer services and worse... I just call it *theft*.

My "time" spent in MBHO was colored indeed by who I was when I entered that business as well. As a native New Yorker I was viewed skeptically to begin with by some Texans. My style of communication is direct and perhaps considered bold, even rude by some. I was unaware of the unspoken rule that my words required sugar coatings and that I had to be a politician. I was instead going with the honesty and forthrightness that was so integrated into my personality. In addition, I had spent ten years as a sole proprietor of my own business at a very early age: I was very good at being a "boss" and making decisions, not so good at *"No see, no hear, no tell"* about so called "rules" too vague to understand. Born and raised in a large extended Italian Catholic family had its influence on how I conducted myself in a business setting as well. Lying, fraud and double standards seemed reprehensible to me, and when it resulted in wasting other people's money, well, that was just plain unconscionable. One could say that I've always been an idealist...

But I was also new to this field, forty something, with a dream. I was anxious to make managed care my last stop in my career. Based on early versions of managed care I was convinced that this was a good fit for me. I just love a challenge that involves trying to **improve** on something. By virtue of the good experiences I had and successes I reached, I knew I could make this my last job before I retire. That was the dream which I persisted in through several managed care plans and companies. My dream began to fall apart after three years, was revived again in the fourth year, and finally crashed after the fifth year. This, despite my persistence and my advocacy for care management and even managed care as a concept.

As a care manager I have witnessed the theft of millions of dollars to pay for fraudulent behavioral health services so providers can line their pockets to fulfill contract obligations. I have also seen services cleverly "diverted" from patients who clearly and clinically needed them to bank up profits for the managed care company. Sadly, I have observed services diluted to save money for all entities involved, and pumped up costs of services to enable insurance companies to profit. I have been privy to the consequences of the deals (contracts) made between the managed care company and some providers–a sort of mutual back scratch–written in obscure language with ever-evolving "updates". These arrangements are not always understood by their own employees and often get miscommunicated. Patients get hurt by these practices. All this, just on my five year watch as an insider working in managed care.

This book is about real life instances of all of the above mentioned offenses. It includes real cases (with changed names to protect identities) with which I personally worked and a diary of the spiritual journey I traveled during these times of intense daily ethical dilemmas in order to keep my job. In the end I hope to convince you that our system can be revised and improved without resorting to socialized medicine.

Diary Entry: Cigna Behavioral Health, 9/03/2000

Medicaid Cesspool

Can't believe they did this to me. 2 awards for care management and I'm stuck in this wasteland. Cases are horrendous. Eleven year olds, eight year olds..., stuck in this hell hole they want to call Residential Treatment Program... It's a ditch—no one even knows her there... they're a factory. Drugs snuck in, kids getting more depressed... They are not even licensed counselors...Is she better off at home with the crazy parents? In today's review they're telling me she is doing great but needs at least 2 more weeks. Two more weeks of what?! Depressed, feeling screwed, betrayed. Should I stay—will they give me a break from these Medicaid cases?? Is there someone I can report this to? It does not seem legal... God hold me up.....

PART II

LEAKS IN THE BOAT

When the author started in this industry in 2000, there was a sense of partnership between the Clinical and the Corporate pieces of the Managed Behavioral Health Care Organization. Care Management was a respectable job and managers and representatives from the corporate office would seek out our feedback and ask us to contribute to their decision making processes. They knew that we knew what was going on and as such had a stake in all processes involving CMs. There was ownership, there was pride, there was a desire to excel and remain a part of this large entity. This was as it should have been. Care managers are the second most educated, trained and experienced in their fields working in managed care next to the doctors.

Yet, their value and special talents gradually became unrecognized and their assessments disregarded. Part II is about the roadblocks to quality care management (and therefore quality health care services) and some of the other significant factors that plague the mental health field in general.

During my tenure as a mental health practitioner I came to realize I did not want to be in a field beleaguered by social and behavioral issues that were regarded as equal to and equally worthy of treatment as mental illnesses. There were never enough funds to treat all these and I believed the seriously mentally ill should take priority. I also found some providers capitalizing on the blurred lines drawn between the mentally ill and the socially maladjusted. In fact, psychiatrists have a category of "personality disorders" which have no medical basis but nonetheless carry hefty sounding titles like "Antisocial Personality Disorder" and "Borderline Personality Disorder" that belie their hopelessly chronic and untreatable nature.

The solution to my complaint about the field appeared very clearly to be managed care. Why here, as an ethical mental health professional, I could make the necessary distinctions and authorize the highest level of care for the really mentally ill while limiting precious resources from the rest of the care seeking population! I could grill the unethical providers and smoke out their greedy motives!   Forever the idealist, I could fix this inequity at last!

This book represents my public confession that I never did beat out the bad guys and right the wrongs, but the field continued to deteriorate instead.

Diary Entry: *Cigna Behavioral Health, 12/15/2000 Moving on?* Today, I asked for some honest answers from the Director of our "care site"; I feel I have earned this much. Michelle tells me I may not be moved from these Medicaid cases, and no, I may not have a raise. That's it. I am done here. It is time for another job hunt. I don't get it: were they lying to me when they gave me these awards for care management? Maybe they just wanted to prevent me from moving up? Lord—I need you...

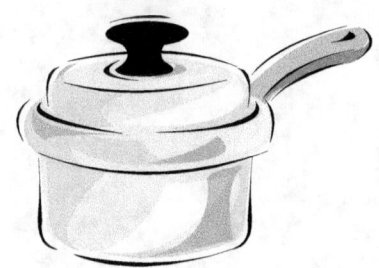

PART II CHAP 1
SQUEEZING OUT THE CARE MANAGER

Unwilling Accomplices in Damaged Care Crimes

Perhaps this industry changed after 911 in 2001, along with many other businesses that were not really solid to begin with. Those interviewed state that the managed care industry fell prey to the gluttonous 90's and over-expanded. Then, when hit with an economic crisis as felt in this country on 911, managed care had to pare down, get lean, cut the waste. It's unfortunate for all of us that it became that obese, and then resorted to such an unhealthy diet!

Those of us who diet know that we should not be cutting out the vegetables and protein first. But that is exactly what these shortsighted bigwigs did. They cut back on their most essential team members, care managers, now operating more like robots who would fall in line with standardized templates and high case loads leaving no time to discuss what is not working or to offer solutions. These care managers are hardly finished completing these sterilized templates when up out of their cubes they sprint to ask their sergeant-supervisor if it is "ok to authorize" this case or that. If it is an HMO they are often told

"NO", (or often "Hell NO!") and directed to send it to Peer Review which will tie up the care manager in a twenty to thirty minute techno-frenzy of red tape until some doctor predictably denies the authorization. If it is a PPO, the care manager will authorize it, period, or face the twenty to thirty minute techno-frenzy of red-tape only to have the doctor *approve* it. They are relegated to *queued* telephone systems and intimidated into rushing through important clinical details that can mean the difference between good patient care and ineffective rubber stamp care. Gone are the days when this author reviewed the case, made an independent decision, consulted with colleagues or called a doctor by phone or took the time to walk into his/her office to chat about a case. Gone are the days when the author was encouraged by supervisors: "You've got to do what you think is best". Gone are the days when the Peer Review was the care manager's option and tool. It has become, well, just another template. This author is willing to bet that doctors miss the old consultations with care managers as well, or they are also mindless robots. And gone are the days, when the care manager can go home and feel proud of the decisions made on the cases of a particular day.

Following are the most damaging obstacles set up for these care managers:

1. **A steady diet of daily ethical dilemmas:**

   Case after case entails real patients with real needs which care managers must continually desensitize themselves to if they want to retain their jobs at the company. Their alternatives in this field are jobs at pay cuts from 30 to 40% These jobs include environments such as private practice, hospitals, private clinics, and non profits..

   Imagine being told to certify additional days for patients who didn't need them or to discontinue hospitalization for patients who desperately need them by someone less trained and experienced than you? This kind of daily humiliation and stress is debilitating and leads to a lack of incentive for doing a good job with each and every case. Eventually, less attention is paid to the details of the case and more attention is paid to pleasing the bosses.

2. **Antiquated technology, multiple computer systems:**

   These are not designed for the care manager to obtain clinical information and complete their goals but for the goals of umpteen others, such as the insurance carriers, the claims department, the Claims department, etc. Care managers used as information gatherers for the statistical needs of regulatory boards, CEOs and the government is another waste of time and money. The pay is good, except if time is spent in mundane busy work which frustrates and wears down the care manager.

This CM, an analytical thinker, was forced to become a multi-tasker, answering phones while inputting information into a computer like a mindless puppet. Technology skills became *more important* than training and education in the mental health field. Logic defied the use of these otherwise magical machines as albatrosses around the care managers' necks, when they were supposed to be tools for efficiency. Some programs had a "glitch" that erased all notes if the CM took more than ten minutes to type them. What is this, sadism?!

Diary Entry: Magellan, Aetna 9/29/01 Brain Pain

Brain Pain—the only way to describe it...low self esteem, constant shame, guilt, confusion, anger, and blaming God. Aetna is trying to kill us—they must want us all to quit! Just when I thought I had a handle on my job, managers talking about increasing case loads, bringing in a new program., more retraining... like the 2000 Aetna screens are not enough...page after page of information gathering while I'm trying to work and document these cases... What do I look like—a data entry clerk...????

Adding insult to injury, programs were continually changing, becoming longer and more complex. As if this was not enough, there were few technicians available for troubleshooting and fixing the machines we were so dependent upon.

3. Chaotic work conditions:

Managers and supervisors with poor communication or organizational skills were not held accountable, as their real function was to pressure care managers. Respect gave way to humiliation of care managers who were not following the company mantra. Blundering through these poorly designed systems of management and then accepting the blame for the inevitable consequences contributed to high turnover among CMs and more disorganization . Newbies endured "shotgun" (and shoddy) training. Morale was excessively low, and most CMs I knew were on some type of medication themselves for depression and/or anxiety. Lists of regulations were ever-changing and requiring updates that were not forthcoming. Cheat sheets of "codes" were constantly undergoing some changes which some of us got and some of us did not. We were notified via e-mail, via flyer, via word of mouth, but never consistently so we were not all on the same page. Systems and procedures were also in a constant state of flux. Memos circulated non-stop about some senate bill or other. I always compared it to working in an ER. What is happening now is changing and what we will do next is unpredictable. We were mental health workers in a dysfunctional environment... At times I wondered if I should pursue unionization for us but I barely had the energy to endure the job as it was. Each night I would come home drained, anxious and demoralized.

3. Conflict of interests with managed care goals:

Care managers became more aware that their services were subjugated to the bottom line principles of profit making over service orientation. Though most CMs are licensed and must adhere to professional guidelines by virtue of that license, we were put in compromising positions and vulnerable to the loss of license for adhering to the mandates of the workplace. As stated earlier, there are alternative work situations for CMs, but the fact remains that only CMs can do what they do. Someone trained and knowledgeable has to manage the many cases before us, consult with doctors, make recommendations for patients and be ultimately responsible for the outcome of the cases. Doctors and Psychologists who are higher up on the pay scale are the only other staff qualified to do the CM's job. In time, objective assessment gave way to filling in generalized intake forms. Providing responsible, good care for patients in turn gave way to following dictates from corporate managers. Keith Dixon, president and CEO of Cigna Behavioral Health writes wonderful articles about that MBHO's successes.

But, the following Memo from "corporate" speaks for itself.

MEMO FROM KEITH DIXON, CEO TO CARE MANAGERS

Interoffice Memo

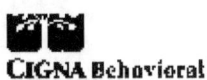

CIGNA Behavioral

Date: September 20, 2004

To: All CBH Employees

From: Keith Dixon

Telephone: 952.996.2120

Facsimile: 952.996.2659

Subject: **Direction on Medical Trend in 2005**

We have been experiencing a medical trend of 12.9% this year. This is not much of an improvement from prior years. This trend level is not acceptable, and will not be supported long term in the marketplace. We need to change it.

As many of you know, I have established a medical trend target of less than 5% for 2005. This is a big challenge. However, it is an achievable goal. We will achieve this through a combination of favorable unit cost execution (e.g. rate negotiations with providers and strategic use of our most cost-effective providers) and utilization. I am relying on the professionalism of our entire clinical community to achieve this result. This is the benchmark on which we will measure our performance in network relations and clinical operations.

A key to success is clear leadership and accountabilities, and disciplined adherence to care management standards and procedures at all sites. In short, we need focused, consistent execution of our Care Advocacy model -- everywhere -- and we need to avoid the temptations of "experimentation" and distractions when things heat up. By now, we all know what to do and how to do it. Everyone needs to stay very focused. To help with discipline and focus, I am making some changes that will help the company align its clinical resources on the tasks at hand.

Effective immediately, all physicians employed or under contract who are working in the Regional Care Centers will report up to Doug Nemecek. All physicians employed by or under contract at the NCC will report up to Craig Coenson. Doug and Craig will now report directly to Jodi Aronson Prohofsky, and indirectly to Rhonda Robinson Beale for issues pertaining to quality. We expect all physicians to stay primarily focused on their support of our care management teams in the RCCs and the NCCs.

Jodi, working in equal partnership with Julie Vayer, owns the 2005 medical trend result at the senior leadership level in the company. Strategic and tactical direction on all matters influencing our medical trend resides with Jodi and Julie. Rhonda will be devoting her considerable talents and energies in 2005 to Quality and Integration -- two huge challenges for us in 2005. Accordingly, Jeff Rubin will now report directly to Rhonda for his work on integration with CIGNA, and I expect him to contribute his operational expertise as needed to our Quality agenda as well as a part of Rhonda's team. We also need Rhonda to lead us in the area of public policy and public affairs in mental health, an arena that will increasingly affect our business. Rhonda, therefore, is the chief external spokesperson for CBH on mental health policy issues.

What these changes are expected to help accomplish is alignment and clear accountability for results in areas of the company that are critical to our success. I expect everyone to be supportive, and to help in every way to get the job done.

It should be obvious to the reader how the care manager was expected to curtail or limit utilization. Since unplugging the phones or eliminating one third of the policyholders were not options, CMs were expected to discourage continued coverage (through Doctor Review) for patients who may have needed it. This is more than unethical and should be illegal.

As the only real personal link to the patient and the only means by which the managed care company can operate its business, one would think that the care manager would be placed in a position of respect or at least some importance in the managed care theater. But while care managers are the folks with the most responsibility they have been stripped of autonomy and morale by the managed care company.

The pot thickens...

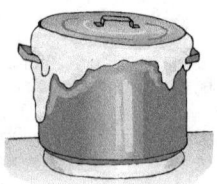

Diary Entry: Magellan, Aetna 3/22/03 Brain Pain

Nothing is as it was since Rick left (former President). He was so creative, so fond of care managers. He walked the floor, stopped to talk to us individually and treated us like professionals. I remember his President's Breakfasts; he'd invite a few of us each month to sit and chat about what we are experiencing on the front line, what we are hearing and seeing in our members and their opinions. The monthly contests were the best. Employees could submit solutions to existing problems and get a monetary reward if the solution was chosen as the best one! My brain hurts—there's fear, anxiety, even paranoia. I think Aetna hates us; they are trying to get us to quit. The screens are increasing—I can't get through them. I'm there 10-12 hours trying to get all my notes in by the skin of my teeth. Uptight, insecure—all dreams dashed...

Part II Chap 2

REGULATION STRANGULATION & BUREAUCRATIC WASTE:

Standardization, The Dysfunctional Family & Communism

The frequent cries to nationalize health care and then pass a law about it so that it is completely funded by the government (your taxes) is frightening when one understands the effects of just *some* of the regulations already in place.

In this section we explore just what the business of managed care looks like when saddled with government interference, URAC, ERISA, HIPAA, HEIDIS, various Senate Bills and the well meaning Patient Bill of Rights Act. Stay tuned for MORE Alphabet Soup...

URAC

URAC DEFINITION: *Utilization Management is the evaluation of the medical necessity, appropriateness, and efficiency of the use of health care services, procedures, and facilities under the provisions of the applicable health benefits plan; sometimes called "utilization review."* (URAC,2001)

In addition to the MBHO's standards for serving patients, URAC defines adequate services to patients as well. As stated earlier there are reams of papers, reports, lists, procedures, current updates, blah, blah, blah. The decision to allow a patient access to services which they believe they are already entitled to by virtue of paid premiums and co-pays is called Utilization Review or UR. In this instance UR is a process as well as the title of the care manager who conducts a review to determine if there is "medical necessity" for a particular service to a particular patient/policyholder. During UR, the CM telephonically reviews symptoms and history as well as the current living situation of each patient and applies the DSM (Diagnostic &Statistical Manual) definitions to these and reviews the policy for coverage. (See also *Definitions*, Part I, Chap 2) Then treatments for the condition are considered carefully in terms of what is best for the individual patient (and what is covered). This utilization review (UR) takes place as frequently as every other day for a patient currently in the hospital, to as infrequently as once per month for a patient who is seeing an out patient therapist. The review commonly involves the care manager at the MBHO and the UR at the provider's office or facility. The patient is rarely consulted about their own symptoms or progress or needs. This is necessitated by the nature of the population we serve. They are in treatment because some part of their mental functioning is not operating adequately. Hello? Contrary to popular belief, care managers *do not* do phone therapy; rather they facilitate the patient's treatment. URAC is an "independent" organization founded in the 1980s because the public was concerned about quality of care and fairness in making such decisions during the course of utilization review (UR). URAC's ultimate purpose is to accredit organizations like the MBHOs who are following their standards for making treatment decisions. With this "accreditation", the MBHO can advertise their greatness. It sounds impressive, it sounds fair, it sounds like the public can trust a company with URAC accreditation.

That said, let's eyeball some of the regulations of URAC:

1. Decisions must be made within two business days of receipt of patient's clinical information.
2. Decisions not to certify must be communicated within one business day to all parties involved
3. Written notification of non-certification must be sent to all parties within one business day. (p 3)

Imagine dozens of cases being managed like individual time bombs by a pool of anxious care managers attempting to meet the time restrictions within the short hospital stay? The clock begins once the care manager is informed that a member has been admitted to a facility for treatment according to another regulation in this section and the rest is havoc within the cubicles of the multitasking care managers.

Since a typical hospital stay (in the managed care world) is three to five days, the race is on to get clinical information about the admission, certify the stay or send the case to Peer Review for possible denial of the stay (CMs are not permitted to deny treatment even if there is no need for it) and then notify all parties before the patient discharges!

The MBHO gains URAC accreditation through scheduled visits in which URAC representatives review their policies and procedures through case files. Trust me, anyone can pass one of these URAC reviews. Care managers always knew when a visit from URAC was expected because supervisors and managers gleaned the case files for the ones that were "clean"–the ones that met the URAC standards. These were placed at the top of the box because it was expected that the "inspector" would quit after reviewing ten or so cases. This loophole was fixed as it became obvious that MBHOs were setting themselves up to pass with flying colors. Next, URAC asked for case files for random dates of operation in an effort to get an accurate assessment of the cases. How do you suppose the MBHOs responded to this? The author will leave this to the reader's imagination. Further inhibiting fairness, URAC's board members are comprised of an array of "experts" such as employers, providers, managed care CEOs, insurance companies and supposedly "the public", but there are no *real insiders* such as care managers on these committees! Not only are CMs left out at the MBHO, they are not welcomed at URAC either. As an illustration, the author attempted to make a report in the form of a complaint to URAC and was referred to my very own employer to make the complaint for me! It's a racket!

TDI

Each state imposes its own regulations on care management. This author is familiar with Texas Department of Insurance through training as a care manager and will describe some of the obstacles set up at Texas MBHOs.

1. Adverse determinations (denials) must go out within one business day
2. Written notices must go to the facility, the provider and the member within one business day.
3. MBHO must not compensate CMs based on lengths of stay or denials.
4. For emergency admissions, CMs will provide decision within one hour of learning that patient is at facility.
5. Medical Necessity Criteria must be applied in a flexible way. (TDI, 2005)

Let's get real. #1,2 and 4 are not doable without adequate technology and/or additional staff to handle notifications.

#3 is a pipedream; managers pressure care managers continuously about their decisions, even giving out report cards of number of denials and lengths of stay for cases handled. As for #5, Medical Necessity Criteria is applied flexibly–by managers, while care managers are often expected to apply them so that the desired outcome is a denial.

NCQA

The Soup turns. NCQA also accredits MBHOs for following *its* standards for patient care. Gaining NCQA accreditation is a status symbol for managed care companies allowing for positive advertising to the public. Sure, there is overlapping with what other regulatory entities do, but what's another regulatory body in a field overwhelmed with regulations?

1. Life threatening conditions: members to be seen within one hour.

2. Non-life threatening but still emergency: members must be seen within 6 hours.

3. Urgent Care: must be seen within 48 hours

4. Routine Office Visit: seen within 10 days

5. Criteria for approvals or denials clearly defined

6. Concurrent review decisions within one working day
7. Non certification (denials) decisions rendered within one day

8. Assists in transition of care when benefits end.

9. Evaluation of technology with input from appropriate professionals

10.Clinical judgments must be made by licensed professionals

11.Cases must be overseen by licensed psychiatrist.

12. MBHOs must monitor under and overutilization of services to members.

(NCQA and Quality Improvement, training provided at Magellan Behavioral Health, 2003).

Let's review: # 1,2, and 3 present some issues. Though this care manager was present when "life threatening" conditions, "non-life threatening but emergency" conditions and "urgent" conditions were defined, I recall that the delineations were quite hazy. Despite this, the time constraints are unrealistic, particularly in some geographical locations where services are few and far between. In #5 the matter of criteria for approval of treatment is handed back to the managed care company, which is like putting the fox in charge of the chicken coup. Now, #6 and 7 are standard, necessitated by the need to know if treatment will be covered by the insurance company as early as possible. But make no mistake about it, meeting these time constraints is most likely when the treatment is *approved*. This is so because *non approval* must be sanctioned by a doctor, (through a Peer Review) and as mentioned previously, is time consuming and tedious. Therein lies the mixed messages given to care managers; deny as much as possible but sending the case to a doctor for that denial will make it harder to comply with regulations–for which we get fined! Yes, some breaches of regulations (that cannot be covered up) cost the managed care company large monetary fines.

ERISA

ERISA is a federal law that regulates *private* healthcare. What? Yes, the government puts its unclean hands into this soup repeatedly. The Employee Retirement Income Security Act of 1974 (ERISA) *does not* attempt to regulate public healthcare such as State or Federal plans or plans established for nonresident aliens or indigent populations. No, no, no; instead, it sets minimum standards and requirements *for plans that cover the employees who voluntarily purchase health care through their employers in private companies.* Among other requirements, it stipulates that:

> "...the companies that manage the plan's funds avoid conflicts of interest when making investment and benefit decisions", that MBHOs "...manage such funds for the "...*exclusive benefit*" of plan participants and beneficiaries", and "...provides that benefit plans must be operated in a fair and financially sound manner". (Hellinger &Young, 2005, p 1)

It is doubtful that today's managed care companies "avoid conflicts of interests" in any way. Their operation involves making treatment decisions and holding the purse strings for treatment simultaneously. So much for that! As for the stipulation that funds are managed for the "exclusive benefit" of plan participants, that may work for non profits but too many managed care companies are in it for profit–big profit.

Other protections include equal benefits to all employees no matter what their medical conditions or disabilities. I am sure readers know someone who has been denied coverage for pre-existing conditions. As long as the laws allow private companies such as Fortis and others to cherry pick their members, a segment of the working population is unprotected. They make too much to qualify for Medicaid but are not covered by their employers. Self employed folks encounter this issue. Does the new law address the self employed?

ERISA regulations are supposedly enforced after an employee obtains a healthcare plan. Enforced how? Employers are free to hire whom they choose, and do not have to offer the healthcare benefits at all to employees. Benefits *do not have to go into effect at the time of employment*. Wait periods for health benefits to kick in can be anywhere from one month to one year. More regs equals more unprotected members.

One supposed benefit of ERISA is that members can now sue their managed care companies for losses arising out of denied coverage for treatment. Hellinger and Young (2005) surveyed laws which allow employees to sue their health care plans to learn what their impact was. They report that ERISA (1974) supersedes state law, and legal cases under this law are heard in *federal court*. For example, the authors report cases against Aetna Health Inc and CIGNA Health Care of Texas in 2004 were preempted at the State level by ERISA.

In other words, ERISA allows for law suits to be brought against the MBHO by policyholders. But the fine print states that these cases have to be brought before the *Supreme Court and not prosecuted at the State level where most consumer complaints originate*. Cases before federal court may only retrieve the monetary cost of the treatment denied, not "mental anguish" or subsequent treatments needed because the original treatment was denied. It seems that for every so called "protection" for the consumer, there is a loophole for MCOs and MBHOs to come out ahead of the consumer.

According to Tom Miller, 2001 director of health policy studies at the Cato Institute:

> The use of..."vague, undefined terms and weasel words ...inevitably would expand bureaucratic discretion and federal micro management through future rounds of reinterpretation,...and "provide the

foundation for lawsuits based on alleged violations of mandatory standards. (Miller, 2001, p 1)

HIPAA

The first federal privacy standards to protect patients' medical records and other health information provided to health plans, doctors, hospitals and other health care providers took effect on April 14, 2003. It was developed by the Department of Health and Human Services.
(Office of Civil Rights, 1996)

Since then it has been difficult for care managers, gatherers of sensitive information, to do their jobs or for parents to find out about their children's treatment, and even for researchers to work on advances in behavioral science.

HIPAA agreements are available in all providers' offices and are generally jammed into patients' hands routinely upon filling out their medical information forms. This act provides rights and protections for participants and beneficiaries in group health plans. It includes protections for coverage under group health plans that limit exclusions for preexisting conditions, and prohibits discrimination against employees and dependents based on their health status. (April 2003). So if an employer knows that a policyholder's dependent child has cancer, health coverage cannot be denied to that particular employee. Does this sound familiar? It should; HIPAA overlaps with ERISA; redundancy and overkill are prevalent in the health care industry.

The MBHO staff undergoes yearly training in these regulations. Ongoing training is necessary because there are some nuances to HIPAA. For example, another right under HIPAA is that employees can continue with healthcare coverage even after they no longer qualify for the benefits, such as loss of job. It should be noted however, that continued coverage, referred to as COBRA, is very expensive and time limited. Most people who lose their jobs probably cannot afford COBRA as stated earlier in this book.

Another protection afforded by HIPAA is privacy regulations for policyholders' health status, whether medical or mental. Patients have control over their health information and can choose who and where this information can be shared by signing these agreements, da, da, da. Of course the information has to be shared with your insurance company and managed care company and all those intake workers and care managers and associated organizations who review your case. Don't believe for one minute that cases are not discussed in less than professional terms. As a health care consumer, this author has received more than one bill in someone else's name complete with personal information about them. Given what the reader has learned about the complexity of the health care industry, "privacy" is doubtful.

When HIPAA is not trying to "protect" policyholders, it is out there making case management complicated. This occurs frequently in cases of seriously mentally ill patients who do not participate or consent to treatment. The author has encountered cases of involuntary patients where the UR (facility CM) could not communicate to the MBHO CM that a patient has a drug history or is on multiple medications because the patient did not sign the HIPAA release form. As a result, the author could not make recommendations for the patient without this significant information and once again "patient care" was compromised. Nice reg. When information cannot pass freely between these two managers of the patient's case, patients are not well served.

Despite the value of HIPAA, according to a survey published in JAMA, researchers must obtain written consent to look at patients' medical records, making it more difficult and costly. In this survey of 1,527 researchers, 70% found the HIPAA laws an impediment to their work while only 25% felt that the law protected the privacy of patients. When privacy protection regulations function as barriers to quality care, the government is quick to pass it but unable to anticipate the consequences. (JAMA, 2008)

Now, cousin FERPA applies specifically to students in educational institutions. The Family Educational Rights and Privacy Act protects the privacy of the health status of students. When HIPAA and FERPA get together, look out! Entanglements with these two can be messy. CMs need yet another regulation and another floating memo. The memo informed care managers that the word "HIV" will no longer be permitted with regard to underage patients when communicating with the school system. No, we were now to use the term "blood dyscrasia", because "HIV" is discriminatory and may interfere with FERPA laws. Within the school system, teachers may not be informed of a high school student's history of mental illness and "hobby" of making bombs in his basement, according to FERPA. At the college level, I will not be informed of a student's mental health issues, including learning disabilities unless the student him/herself informs me. These are not protections; they are obstacles.

Entitlements

Title V funds, which come out of SSA (Social Security Act) benefit children with special needs and/ or low income status. Title XIX established Medicaid which is financed by the state and federal government out of "general revenues", otherwise known as *your taxes*. Since many MCOs and MBHOs now manage at least some of Medicaid and Medicare, more overlapping regulations must be implemented (and memorized) by the CM. The author is especially reminiscent of the CIGNA cases of Medicaid children stowed away in the RTCs while they were "benefitted" by Title XIX and Title V funds...

The funds did not cover oversight by a medical doctor nor did the managed care company provide one to the care manager– many of these places are rat holes...

JCAHO and More...

Would you like to be Joint Commission compliant? These regulations apply to hospitals and patients receiving care at hospitals. Since MBHOs admit patients to hospitals these regulations become our business as well. Considering admitting a patient to a non JCAHO hospital? CMs may not claim ignorance and will be chastised for sending a patient to such a facility. JCAHO certification? Sure, let's have another endorsement. There are *many* more regulations on care management in this industry but the author has selected to end the torture here for brevity's sake.

Case In Point #1: BCBS 5/02/03, Regulation Strangulation

Jason Hines, 14, was admitted to a residential treatment program (RTC) on 12/6/03 with a diagnosis of 304.03, Cannabis Dependence. This facility has a reputation for admissions that don't meet criteria and UR tend to be manipulative and poorly educated. Jason was brought in by his parents after having been found smoking marijuana. Patient reports smoking five joints per day for the last two years. His toxin screen is positive for cocaine as well. The patient reports use of cocaine on weekends with last use two weeks ago. Vitals are normal and doctor's notes indicate no symptoms of withdrawal. There are no medical or physical conditions requiring special care. Patient has no previous admissions or attempts at treatment of any kind. Mental status is normal, no suicidal, homicidal or psychotic features. Patient's grades are poor but passing, reports some mild symptoms of depression: poor appetite and sleep, less activity. There are no legal charges current except for suspension from school for possession last year. Ordered medications: Zoloft 50.

CM is asking for more information before making determination but the UR does not have it. Regular reviewer is on another case and doctor left for another facility. Providers often expect an approval without giving all the information needed to give an approval.

LOOK OUT! REGULATION: URAC

URAC mandates that the care manager will accept information from "any reasonably reliable source", and collect only information necessary to certify admission, treatment or length of stay, and base decisions solely on information obtained at the time of the review.

Essentially, the care manager is being told not to think...

At this time there is incomplete information to indicate this admission is medically necessary thanks to the lower standards for providers imposed by URAC. It should be noted that the RTC facility UR are not held to the same standards as CMs at the MBHO. The CM has two choices: approve this admission even though it does not seem warranted, or send the case to Peer Review for the doctors to discuss the case and make a determination. Oh no! Not another Peer Review!

LOOK OUT! REGULATION: NCQA

CM has 24 hrs to let the facility know determination and deliver letters to patient, facility and attending doctor. Get going! It's 2pm!

Completing Rationale for Peer Review:

First, attach all clinical information gathered in the initial review. This is done the "cut and paste" way of course. Attach copy of Medical Necessity Criteria for RTC admission for 14 year olds because we can't be bothering our doctors with these details. (cut and paste again). Since CM is recommending a lower level of care, it is protocol to call around to see which one might be logistically feasible and have an opening. Again, this involves phone calls and endless documentation into the lame computer program. Justification for denial of RTC admission: more information is needed about family and how supportive they are to treatment. For example: Is anyone else in the house using? Does patient and guardian have access to a car and a less intensive treatment option other than the RTC? Is there any history of depression or suicidality in the family? Patient does not seem to meet criteria for RTC admission. Here we go: more documentation both into program and onto a Peer Review Request Form. Think we're done? NOT! It's 2:45pm

Next call the Peer Review Request Line to get the review scheduled. But wait! This procedure has recently been "updated"; now we can e-mail the Peer Review Request Team! E-mail, cut and paste, cover page, policy number, case type number, this code, that code, hit the wrong button and everything is lost... Well, this does take the case out of the CM's hands, right? NOT, again! Sending this colossal dissertation to the bachelor level clerks has its disadvantages. Generally, they do not understand a word of its content but will promptly "assign" it to the appropriate doctor to review: " Let's see now is it Dr Blue who specializes in multiple substance abuse or Dr Red who specializes in multiple personality disorder?...." This decision is not placed in the hands of the care manager of course because what do they know? Now it is 3:15pm.

LOOK OUT! REGULATION: HIPAA

Members' names or other identifying information (ss#) may not be used in order to protect members' privacy. E-mail to the Peer Review Request Team must not contain the name or social security number of the policyholder. They will have to figure out who this is through *their* inadequate technology! The Team is requesting we send them the file to make their jobs easier, and because the doctor will make his notes inside the case. Since they are positioned five yards away, CM will *walk* the file to the Peer Review Request Team, after sending the information laden e-mail to them *without the patient's name* requesting the peer review. It should be clear to the reader that a less meticulous CM would "just authorize it", a lazy CM would "just authorize it", a robot would "just authorize it". Perhaps most others would "just authorize it". As a conscientious professional it appears that Peer Reviews and carpal tunnel retirement are my destiny.

LOOK OUT! REGULATION: TDI

All parties must receive written communication of the outcome within 24 hours.

If and when the "determination" (decision) from the doctors comes back in time (after overcoming schedule obstacles), the next leg of the race is on. It starts with another inefficient process for getting all the letters out before the 2pm deadline – the Letter Request Form. This is a tremendous improvement over the days when the care manager had to actually type each letter on the non user-friendly computer program!

Since there are around twenty cases on a typical care manager's caseload, chances are 15% or more of them are in Peer Review simultaneously. When providers give inadequate information, make poor medication choices, provide substandard care, or fail to produce a logical discharge plan, there will be Peer Reviews requested by the care manager all day long. How else can we *manage* the cases with integrity?

So this was the thinking: Take the burden off the care manager, streamline the process, standardize it, and regulate it all at the same time! Let's see now... The care manager calls the scheduler who then calls the facility asking for the scheduler/ur person/ representative for the doctor to schedule their doctor to speak with our doctor. As Murphy's Law would have it, the UR line is busy, the provider's doctor is not at the facility, and the MBHO doctor is booked for the rest of the day. It's 4pm...

Waynette will schedule this Peer Review when she gets in the next day at 8am. The CM is SO motivated now to wake up to the next morning's alarm. Not, not, not...

Diary Entry: BCBS, 4/15/03 Still a Newbie...

Dipped real low   at work today–it's that damn pager–the uncertainty, the "sitting duck" feeling–being ready on command.   Heck, I don't even answer my phone at home if I don't feel like talking...but here I am, already an over-anxious ball of nerves, on hyper alert.   So in the meantime, I go and get lost in some

P.A. screens, leading me on a wild goose chase, when here comes Maryanna–I call her "Lucy" –as in "Lucy & Desi", looking at me incredulously like "YOU SHOULD KNOW THIS STUFF"–I am already down some brain cells secondary to depression but she's got me crawling on the floor with the lowest forms of life!   She just has that way of acting like she thinks I'm stupid!   Give me a break...I just started –coming from   an entirely different Team.....

Part II CHAP 3

STAT!

Templates & Qs & Time Tracking, Oh my!

The Templates

Now, here comes the industry's version of keeping order in the behavioral health world: TEMPLATES!   That's it! We'll just round up all these patients and their information into neat little TEMPLATES!!   Heavy standardization is a practice currently being used within MBHOs. It is probably a great idea for simple tasks such as buying tires or stamps. Proponents of templates point to its value for information gathering. Templates are heavily used in the field of education to assess, evaluate, measure knowledge, ability and so forth. But when applied to a population of mentally ill people –not so much!   As stated several times in this book, the generally unstable, unpredictable patients are often in crisis. They miss their follow up appointments, abruptly suspend their medications, admit to the hospital at odd hours of the night, have splintered families or no families, they may not be able to drive, and they are incoherent half of the time.   As an illustration of what the practice of standardization is really like applied to this population, try to imagine putting them on an automated telephone system:

> "If you are in crisis press 1, if you feel suicidal press 2, if you just took an overdose of lethal pills, press 3....."
> You get the picture.

This standardization of practices and procedures also shuts out the CM who has the training, education and judgment to gather information and make decisions for patients. Standards have improved medical health care, but not mental health care. Follow up care after hospitalization and integration of services for patients still fail to meet quality levels. (Moran, 2004) Moran asks: are health plans doing anything "to provide incentives or make it easier for clinicians (CMs) to meet the performance measures"? (p 5) The answer is 'no'; they are instead setting up an obstacle course for care managers.

Case In Point #2: BCBS 6/12/03 Prader Willi Disease

Matthew M, twelve year old male, admitted to psychiatric facility following fourteen days in an RTC (Residential Treatment Center), where he was constantly in restraints and seclusion. He was therefore stepped up to inpatient level of care. Diagnosed "Mood Disorder Not Otherwise Specified", 296.90, ADHD and Intermitted Explosive Disorder. Patient has an extensive previous history of multiple hospitalizations; this is his third admission in the last month alone. Symptoms include aggression, attacking others, throwing and destroying items, poor relationships with others. Mother states patient has been this way since birth. Patient has low frustration level, low grade depression, misjudges social situations, goes into unprovoked rages. Patient also eats constantly, is obese, has a family history of schizophrenia and mental retardation. Mother reports she cannot contain him at home and previous treatments have had no effect on him.

This poor youngster had no testing after having been in an RTC for fourteen days, three hospitalizations, and several months at a State Facility in the last six months alone. CM ordered a transfer to a facility that can administer testing. The following was required to accomplish this goal:

1. research and multiple phone calls to hospitals that can test,
2. another template for a transfer,
3. a doctor to doctor review (Peer Review),
4. a template for the review, multiple phone calls to set it up,
5. documentation of doctor's determination which is a denial of continued stay at the current facility and admission to new facility.

6. template for sending letters to parties involved about denial determination and verbal notification to all parties (NCQA, TDI regulations)

7. notification of approval of admission to all parties for new facility.

8. submission of forms to psychologist requesting specific tests such as an EKG, psychological and neuro-psychological testing.

9. continued reviews while patient undergoes testing at new facility.

10. documentation of all of the above into the tired computer program.

This long delayed testing revealed the patient has mild MR (mental retardation), IQ score 72, and Prader Willie disorder, a rare, genetic medical condition causing insatiable appetite and uncontrolled outbursts in response to intense frustration. CM now had to send this case to doctor review again to transfer patient to long term care while he receives medication. This, because the current facility will not voluntarily discharge this patient without a formal denial and a formal determination that his condition is "organically" driven (medical) not mental. Torte reform anyone?

The parent also required help applying for disability and Medicaid for this child's treatment. More forms, more telephone calls, more letters, more regulations, more time waste... When it was all over this patient was traumatized and his mother was exhausted. Admittedly, he finally had a proper diagnosis and appropriate medicines for his condition. One wonders why this could not be done sooner, why previous facilities had not attempted to test this fourteen year old. And especially, why the process was so tedious... "Managed" care? I don't think so.

It is the height of ridiculousness when Master's level care managers are being given TEMPLATES to use with which to gather information when gathering information is what we have been trained to do! The author is not talking about name, address and telephone number here; anyone can do that kind of information gathering. Whether we are talking on the telephone with a facility representative, entering the clinical information into a computer, or giving the info to a consulting doctor, the confining TEMPLATE dictates the questions, the order in which to ask them, and even the space allowed for acceptable answers! Sometimes, the template even contains a limited selection of multiple choice type questions and answers most of which do not apply to the current case. Readers can imagine what it would be like if the CIA and FBI agents were given templates to complete their interrogations!

Case In Point #3: Magellan Aetna 2/19/03
History of Substance Abuse

Miriam W. is a 32 year old female who is a frequent flyer to the hospital circuit. Diagnosed with Bipolar Disorder and Substance Abuse, she has a history of suicidality and criminal behaviors around drugs. She alternates between jail for drug related charges and hospitalization for suicidality. Miriam has a total of 11 hospitalizations in the past 14 years, three so far this year. Her father attempts to keep her at home to monitor her treatments, medications and drug use but Miriam leaves for days at a time without notice. She has no other support. CM is determined to do something different with this patient and reviews previous hospitalizations, medications used, discharge plans, etc. CM then calls the UR at the admitting facility for an initial review. UR Patty at the Happy Face Psychiatric Facility reports that Miriam has been diagnosed with Bipolar Disorder and was given Clozaril 125mg, Resperdol 2, Valium 10, Xanex and Ativan as needed. Patient is uncooperative, labile and refusing to attend groups. **Patient denies any substance abuse** issues, is suicidal and has not signed a release of information at this time.

CM has information from previous hospitalizations that this patient has a substance abuse history and therefore should not be on any drugs that are addicting such as Valium, Xanex and

Ativan. However, CM was unable to inform Patty of previous hospitalizations, history of substance abuse and incarcerations due to drug offenses because of ERISA. CM used several tactics to exchange information without violating regulations from asking if a drug screen was done upon admission to suggesting a Peer Review to review the treatment plan. Unfortunately, a Peer Review could not be arranged due to the unavailability of the treating doctor at that time. Miriam will receive the inappropriate medications and probably trigger her drug addiction and she will be back in the hospital next month.

This is not "care"; it's a waste of time, resources and taxpayer monies. And if and when the federal government becomes the new "middle man" it will probably be worse.

My cup of soup runneth over...

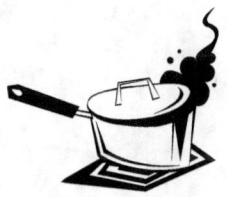

Sample Intake Template:

INITIAL REVIEW

Abbreviation	Long Heading	Needed Content
UR:	UR Contact:	Who, Credentials, Phone and Location (if not hosp UR).
PT:	Patient Information:	Confirm name, age, DOB, address and phone.
AP/FC:	AP/Facility Information:	Date Admitted and LOC (or proposed for preadmit). Specify Network Status of AP and Facility (If OON benefits or adhocs provide details). PCP name, phone number and when contacted
DX:	Diagnosis:	List Axis 1 thru 5 Diagnoses
WHY ADM:	Why Admitted:	Precipitants and why now. Presenting symptoms and mental status. Risk Assessment and History. Judgment/ Other Risk Factor.
TX HX:	Treatment History(CD/MH)	Compliance/What has and had not worked. Barriers and strengths to f/u treatment. Current Use/Abuse (collaborate with CD assessment, family reports, UDS). Current withdrawal symptoms. Dual Dx issues being addressed.
TX PLAN:	Treatment Plan and and LOC/LOS Requested	How going to resolve problems causing admit at this time including medication adjustments, psychotherapies, social support engagement. Discharge/Aftercare Plans (Name/Date/Time).
CM REC:	Care Manager Recommendations:	If days approved: LOC approved, LOC and LOS approved. Cite Rationale, Criteria and Disclaimer Read Any quality of care concerns. If PA Referral: Cite Rationale and criteria not met.. State recommended ALOC and additional issues/questions for PA to address
NEXT:	Next Review:	Date/Time of update. contact person.

By the time all of the items on this form are addressed, the document will be about three pages long. These are extensive documents! Imagine attempting to get this information telephonically while entering same into an inadequate computer program? The technology to improve this system was out there but was not considered important enough to make the investment by the MBHO. This because care managers were expected to be machines themselves, hobbling through with inadequate support. And hobble we did...

Another significant way the TEMPLATE is being used is to send a case for a Peer Review. This is an all important procedure used in the event that the care manager employed by the MBHO and the UR ("utilization reviewer") at a particular provider or facility do not agree about some aspect of the case. Readers are probably unaware that care managers are fighting for them about so many aspects of their treatment by monitoring medications, facility procedures, group and individual therapy sessions, family involvement with the patient, and discharge planning that is customized for the patient. Length of stay disagreements for the patient are the most common reason to request a Peer Review. This is simply a higher level decision made between the MBHO doctor and the doctor caring for the patient (treating doctor). As stated earlier, the form used to request such a review is tedious and time consuming. It is important to remember here that decisions about length of stay between managed care and the provider are time sensitive; they must be determined within twenty four hours of the review itself. Tic, toc.

The idea is to standardize our procedures so that there's less margin for error? I can assure you that after doing a number of these with real live patients, 95% of whom do not fit the template, that the errors are *greater* with the template! In addition, the time wasted improvising so the template will function at least minimally, navigating around its artificial categories, and completing the necessary technology associated with it is time consuming, inefficient and economically wasteful. In summary, we have marginalized the mentally ill population and diluted the clinical picture for patients, leaving questions as to the efficacy of the treatment selected. And, no, the MBHO doctor does not see the patient. This is a good thing?

Another trend and closely related cousin of standardization in managed care, and a throwback to the 1960s is *centralization.* While our country at large is examining the mistakes of the past and recognizing that populations in different locations have cultures and lifestyles that are distinct and require their own set of services and solutions, managed care is into CENTRALIZATION. This is echoed by managers in the frequent statements that begin with: "CORPORATE WANTS US TO...". It distances all employees in a particular office site, from "Corporate", those far away folks who are doing the business piece who generally understand our work as little as we understand theirs. And the disconnect grows and detracts from morale; "We are in it for the patients, They are in it for the money", is a typical employee sentiment.

Diary Entry: BCBS, 4/14/03 The Queue is coming...
Got the news today: we go from a pager to a "Queue" system. The pager was bad enough–not knowing what kind of call will come through. Inpatient care manager was perfect for me; I knew what kind of calls were coming my way and I was prepared. I thought I was doing a good job with that, now... Simple things overwhelm me. Lay down and die, sit down and cry, hide behind the sofa...I want so badly to rise up and beat this but it's an endless pit. My spirit is broken. Oh, God, teach me confidence with humility, speak to me....Is it time to quit?

Like centralization, communism doesn't work either: Check the history books. Most employees at a managed care company are stuffed into cubes and subject to the "Queue" (a mindless phone system described shortly). The caseloads are overwhelming or poorly distributed and staff is shifted at will through "cross training" programs in which the training is poor and the "crossing" is always disruptive for all involved. Upper management never appears to be sensitive to the consequences of these upheavals, just pushes personnel around as needed regardless of job descriptions, interview promises, personal requests, whatever. There's a saying in Texas about the weather: If you don't like it-- wait five minutes. Well, there's a similar saying in managed care: If you don't like it, wait three months. (it will change or even return to the way it was).

Case in Point #4: Magellan, Aetna, 8/27/2001, Nine Lives

Denise O is a 46 year old female admitted to facility with suicidal ideation and a plan following overdose on 30 Trazodone. Found by husband, patient has a history of rape with flashbacks which precipitated the suicide attempt. Clinical information: poor memory, lethargic, weight loss 50 pounds in 6 months, insomnia, no psychosis and oriented to name and time. Patient also has history of one hospitalization, substance abuse-last use unknown. Current medications: Depakote 500 bid, Luvox 100 bid, Ativan .5 q2 hs (every two hours as needed at night), Seroquel 25. Care manager authorizes 6 days with next review 9/2/01, at which time CM will expect more thorough substance abuse history and more information in general.

9/2 Review: Patient is reportedly banging head at night, pacing, having nightmares about gang rape. CM now learning patient had BAL (blood alcohol level) of 226 on admission and admits to consuming a six pack prior to suicide attempt. Patient is on suicide watch Q15 minutes, withdrawn and reclusive, attending 50% of group therapy sessions provided by the hospital. Withdrawal symptoms: diaphoresis, anxiety, agitation, mild tremors, elevated vitals. Current Medications: Depakote 500 bid, Seroquel increased to 100hs, 25am, Ativan 2hs, Ativan .5 bid, added Neurontin 400, 800hs. ("hs"= evening, "am"= morning, "bid"= twice per day).

Care manager note: Patient is on an enormous amount of meds, still detoxing and suicidal after seven days and no family session has taken place to determine actual support at home.

9/2-Care manager requests Peer Review to address meds and length of stay. Care manager spends rest of day preparing forms, notifying scheduler, documenting all clinical and working on the rest of the mounting case load.

9/3-Case went to Peer Review with Dr. A.

9/4- Received result of Peer Review: Did they address all of CM's concerns? No, but the MD retro- authorized 9/3, 9/4, with review on 9/5 for possible discharge.

9/4- Care manager notifies all parties telephonically and by electronic letter of new authorized dates and last covered date. CM documents all in computer as well. (All very time consuming, tedious and repetitive)

9/5 Review: Patient continues to meet medical necessity criteria (MNC) for hospital level of care, still suicidal with plan. Attending physician wants to adjust medications: Adding Topomax and Abilify. Still no family session with husband.

Care manager is concerned that the facility may be helping patient process her rape which is delaying stabilization and should be arranged in long term outpatient counseling or step down to partial hospitalization. However, it is not advisable to discharge over a weekend... so care manager authorized 9/5 through 9/7. Next review 9/8.

9/8 Review: Patient still head banging, angry with husband which is why no family session has taken place. Patient continues with insomnia and not eating, now being given Ensure. Updated meds: Trazodone 200hs,Abilify 15, Ativan 1bid, 2hs, and discontinue Elavil and Topomax. Facility UR asks for six additional days to wrap up work on rape and abuse issues. (Say what?!)

CM is very concerned that this patient is deteriorating, and the attending physician changed meds around again but has not titrated (slowly reduced dosage) down Ativan, (recommended for patients with history of substance abuse). CM is further concerned that the attending MD has lied in his first review with Dr. A, denying that the hospital is processing patient's rape and abuse issues, and facility UR is unclear about patient's psychosis—all Quality of Care issues.

9/8   CM requests Peer Review #2, paperwork, forms, notifications, scheduling, etc and so forth.

9/9 Case goes to another Peer Reviewer with Dr. B.

9/9 Results of Peer Review received at the end of that day. Dr. B denies continued stay, recommending step down to partial hospitalization with continued out patient individual therapy. Since it is the end of the day, the care manager stays late to document results, notify all parties telephonically and by letter of results of Peer Review and denial dates and last covered day.

This patient discharged finally. But due to marital conflicts and continued substance abuse was readmitted to same facility one month later.   In fact, three subsequent hospitalizations occurred for a total of sixty-six (66) days. Included of course were multiple Peer Reviews, paperwork, delays, days authorized due to regulations and continued quality of care issues. It was learned that the patient had "unlimited coverage" so there was no chance of depleting her benefits. Facilities and providers know this—and some unfortunately take advantage of patients by requesting more hospital days. It's another racket. Damaged care, screeching high costs and regulation strangulation were the highlights of this case...

The "Queue"

Now, let's talk about the Queue, ("Q" for short). If you have not experienced this you don't know what you are missing. It's got many variations, but the basic idea is that the phone rings at everyone's desk and it better be picked up in short order by the "next available staff" or else... There's all sorts of surveillance of who picked up the phone how many times and how long it took them to answer and how long they stayed on the phone, etc. This is the model often used for many "call centers". Most of the time, it is used by intake personnel but some managed care companies are trying to impose it on other employees. Here's one activity I wouldn't mind outsourcing, like to Communist China. The new system was named "First Call Resolution", meaning that the caller's issue would be resolved in the same phone call. Imagine how unrealistic it is for managed care companies to implement this system when care managers are already operating in an ER type of environment, with crisis situations and patients who are critically ill and threatening suicide or homicide, and constrained by time tables and regulations? The "Q" is simply unrealistic.

Case in Point #5: Magellan, Aetna 11/30/01,
Too Many Cooks...

One case sent to Peer Review went like this: On 12/1 a call is received from a facility that a patient had admitted on 11/30. His symptoms sounded serious and he met the criteria so he was authorized for that day. But on 12/1 this patients symptoms had resolved and he sounded like he could discharge that day so it was not authorized. Instead it was sent to Peer review. It did not get scheduled until 12/2, at which time the patient discharged.   The scheduler calls the representative for the doctor who then says: "Oh, wait, it says here this patient discharged". Both assume the Peer Review is not needed any longer. So the scheduler calls the care manager to inform her of this but the care manager is out to lunch. She comes back from lunch expecting to see a result from the Peer Review knowing full well there are only two hours left to the 24 hour deadline. Instead she hears the message that the patient discharged. So she calls the scheduler back and says: " I know the patient discharged on 12/2 but the date in question is 12/1. It was not authorized and we may not want to pay for that extra day. Please reschedule this". So scheduler calls the representative for the doctor who is out to lunch. Then, scheduler calls the doctor directly to attempt to reschedule the Peer Review to determine if 12/1 was indeed a necessary hospital day for this patient. Dr. Mess says to the scheduler again: "The patient is discharged and everything has been taken care of" and hangs up! I just want to know: "Who's on first?" !

This is a sneaky way to extract an extra day from the insurance company who is paying for it. No, wait! **We** are paying for it! But the real crime here is the tangled bureaucracy which obscures the reality of what is going on.

And this saga continues until the clock runs out and the day 12/1 had to be authorized because wo, the managed care company, did not schedule the peer review within 24 hours. The care manager handling this case was heavily chewed out and received a "ding" on her evaluation for the incident. What idiot dreamed up this regulation without provisions for the inevitable? Congressmen and women? And who are the bunglers that think this is a good process to insure the regulations are being met? Congressmen and women? And how can this be good patient care? Congressmen and women?

Tic-toc, tic-toc....

But by and far, "Time Tracking" takes the prize for most obnoxious standardization of practices. This program was purchased by Magellan to "help identify our job descriptions" for the purpose of "maximizing our individual potentials" (and provide good documentation for layoffs). My experience with this system ended with a near mental breakdown. Here is how it worked: A cumbersome and awkward program for tracking the employee's use of time on the job is installed on the CMs already user unfriendly and antiquated computer. The program lists the estimated components of the care manager's job, each accompanied by a "fill in the blank" time period to complete each task each day. So for example one task might be "Telephone Call", followed by time started, followed by time completed.

Task #7

Outgoing telephone call   Started: 10:20am   Completed: 10:36am

Task #12

Consultation with MD   Started: 11:00am   Completed: 11:17am

Eventually, "telephone call" came off our list of tasks and Magellan opted to enter a device on our telephones for timing (and tapping!).

At the end of the day, the numbers are tallied and total times are recorded in each task and believe it or not it was actually RATED on a daily basis! The process itself was time consuming and that should have been figured into the total but it was not. Lunch breaks were left out and managers had to recalculate for them. Therefore the figures given at the end were hardly meaningful to CMs–but they were deemed meaningful to our superiors! The tasks themselves were a problem, for whoever created this instrument did not know the job of the care manager! Over the year and a half period that it was used by care managers, it was continuously being overhauled to meet the realities of the care manager position. The items were vague and redundant and many more were missing then were included! The company that sold this bomb to our brilliant CEO did not invite one care manager in the development of the program. My anxiety was at a level I had never known up to this point in my life...

Diary Entry: Aetna, Magellan 11/02/2002,
In Your Dreams...The Dream: This was hilarious. In my dream a coworker received an e-mail about a new procedure about to go into effect called "Situational Management". Like the crappy plans thrown at care managers, this one was meant for managers! The coworker jumped up from her desk in response and gathered other team members around her to commiserate about this news and was overheard whispering frantically: "But I don't think Karen (new President) knows we are going LIVE with "Situational" this Thursday!" Looking somber the group quickly dispersed, no solutions in hand. I sat at my computer shaking my head with a smirk–"That's it!", I thought to myself. Then I woke up just laughing my head off!

The funny part lies in the meanings not dramatized in the dream. It seems that "Situational Management" was the care managers' version of "First Call Resolution"–a turning of the tables if you will. It required that management respond immediately to a care manager who has a question or problem with a case. Typical care manager requests are: "I've spoken to Mrs Smith 26 times today, would you take the next call and explain to her why her son's RTC (Residential Treatment Center) was denied?" Or this one: "Patient's BAL (blood alcohol level) was 462 at admission, must I send this to doctor review or can I just authorize it?" and my personal favorite: "I have 36 cases today. Can I be excused from the "Advanced Care Management" workshop today?"

Under "Situational Management" all managers were to be cross trained across all computer programs, all insurance plans and will know the operations, job descriptions and nuances of each team and how it functions. This should come very naturally to them since they are the "best minds" we have in managed care and can run this place without us. If a team is operating smoothly, why waste that manager's skills with reading magazines or surfing the internet when some desperate care manager on another team needs a manager's help?

The new plan will be rolled out in Wednesday's meeting and will go "live" on Thursday.   Roller skates or sneakers will be appropriate attire for the first week.   I can't wait!

Sample Original Tasks List:

Task definitions assigned to TX Clinical - UM Support group.

General Task	Specific Task	Quantities (Units [RE])
ADHOCS - FACILITY	BCBS (TX)	Total(Requests[15])
ADHOCS - FACILITY	TX RSC	Total(Requests[3.3])
ADHOCS - PROVIDER	BCBS (TX)	Total(Requests[12])
ADHOCS - PROVIDER	TX RSC	Total(Requests[3.3])
AFTER CARE COORDINATION	TX RSC	TBT
AFTER HOURS ADMITS	AETNA (TX)	Total(Cases[6.7])
AFTER HOURS ADMITS	MULTI (TX)	Total(Cases[4.6])
AUTH CORRECTIONS	TX RSC	Total(Cases[5.5])
CASE CONSULTATION	TX RSC	Occurrences(Events[30])
CASE F/U	TX RSC	Total(Cases[6])
CASE MANAGEMENT / REVIEWS (ROUNDS)	TX RSC	TBT
CASE PREP. - URAC	TX RSC	Total(Cases[3])
CASEWORK	TX RSC	Total(Cases[20])
COMPLAINTS / GRIEVANCES	TX RSC	Total(Cases[5.4])
CONCURRENT REVIEW (HIGHER LOC)	BCBS (TX)	Total(Cases[4])
CONCURRENT REVIEW (HIGHER LOC)	TX RSC	Total(Cases[3.2])
CRISIS CALL	TX RSC	Total(Calls[6])
CUSTOMER SVC. CALLS	TX RSC - CLINICAL	Total(Calls[24])
FACILITY TRANSFER	TX RSC	Total(Requests[2])
FAMILY MEMBER CONTACTS	TX RSC	Total(Calls[6])
HEALTH PLAN INTERACTION	TX RCC	Occurrence Events[2]
INDEPENDENT / EXTERNAL REVIEWS	BCBS (TX)	Total(Cases[6])
INDEPENDENT / EXTERNAL REVIEWS	TX RSC	Total(Cases[12])
INDEPENDENT / EXTERNAL REVIEWS F/E	BCBS (TX)	Total(Cases[2])
INITIAL ASSESSMENTS (HIGHER LOC)	BCBS (TX)	Total(Cases[2.4])
INITIAL ASSESSMENTS (HIGHER LOC)	TX RSC	Total(Cases[2])
INTENSIVE CARE MANAGEMENT (ICM)	TX RSC	TBT Total(Calls)

Understand that the care manager, while performing a super multi-tasking job with crisis cases (patients being rushed to psychiatric facilities), was expected to tune in to this Time Tracking program on another screen on the desktop computer, already in use to document the current case, and click on the task currently being performed and how many minutes it takes to complete! You really had to be there...

Supervisors and managers were having their own headaches with the program because they were expected to retrieve our daily "performance ratings" and incorporate them into our assessments. Issues came up about why other employees were not using Time Tracking like doctors, managers, claims workers, etc. But it was never applied to them. This was an absolute abomination perpetrated upon care managers. Many wondered if it was just a tool to select potential layoffs during a time when the company was facing bankruptcy.

Several months after TT (Time Tracking) was installed and in use, management began to see the flaws in the $75,000 program, thanks to the untiring complaints from employees who were required to use it. In addition, some really ingenious individuals figured out how to cheat the system and claim high ratings every day... CMs were livid; some resigned, but I hung in there until I was ragged, fearful, hyper-vigilant and paranoid.

The following e-mail from "corporate" confirms what everyone already knew about this program:

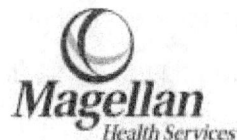

Magellan
Health Services

To: RSC Colleagues
From: Danna L. Mézin
Date: February 12, 2003
Subject: ABI Focus Group Feedback

Last week, CSRs, Care Managers, and Supervisors from RSCs around the country participated in a continuous improvement focus group regarding the Accelerated Business Improvement Initiative (ABI). The participants shared their views on the initiative's key successes and identified improvement opportunities, specifically as they related to the initiative's processes and tools. These views were recorded and presented to me today by the focus group's facilitator, Joann Albright. Two themes emerged from the focus groups:

1. ABI successfully brought focus to our service performance and introduced processes and tools to help team members appreciate and manage their individual and team contributions.

 2. While many of the tools introduced by ABI have proven very effective, there is profound concern that TTS does not meet our needs as a performance measurement vehicle and, in fact, may be creating an obstacle to serving our customers.

It was great to learn that, overall, the group appreciated the value of ABI. However, what drew my attention most was the focus group's passion surrounding concerns as they relate to TTS.

First and foremost, make no mistake; we are a Company firmly grounded in the value and need for every Magellan team member to be accountable for the quality, productivity and impact of his/her work. It is only through measurable goals that we can determine success and be held accountable for our respective contributions. However, measurements must be meaningful, accurate, and, most importantly, drive positive behaviors and results that facilitate goal achievement.

Many of the focus group participants suggested that TTS does not meet our accountability requirements and requested that we consider an alternative measurement approach. This message echoed sentiments that have been shared with me as I have been visiting the RSCs and that have been shared through a variety of other communication channels. In response to the compelling assessment of TTS, over the next week, we will form a cross-functional work group to identify and develop an alternative to the current TTS tool. This work group will include representation from the employee groups that directly use TTS, leadership team members that use TTS metrics as a decision making tool, and technology resources that can help implement an IT-based solution.

My expectation is that this work group will be deliberate in its efforts and that a revised measurement approach recommendation will be defined within the next 30 days and executed as quickly as possible thereafter. In the interim, we will continue using TTS as the basis for many of our performance metrics; however, we will not advance TTS' deployment to locations not currently using the system. To help us make the best go forward decision, I request that every effort be made to use TTS in the spirit that it was intended until such a time that TTS is enhanced to be a more viable tool or an alternative is implemented.

I would like to thank those individuals who participated in the focus group and shared their concerns in an effort to improve our company's performance. Together, we ensure that we all accept accountability for our performance and that the tools we use to determine our success are effective and meaningful

The reasons for the failure of this expensive and ineffective program are similar to the reasons why the Template doesn't work and are the same reasons why over regulation does not work, particularly with the mentally ill population and in the atmosphere of crisis in which care managers operate. Could you imagine emergency room staff "time tracking" their activities? How about police officers confronting criminals? Patients entering psychiatric hospitals following a complex suicide attempt fit the same descriptions. The situation is fluid—split decisions are made, multitasking is going on and more than one services or treatments are being applied, not to mention the never ending reactions from managers, and the constant fear of litigation. Not surprisingly, the diligent, dutiful and honest CM would choose quality of care in imminent and volatile situations over entering numbers correctly into a computer. Inadequate data entry will be held against the care manager and may lead to dismissal. Been there, done that.

Diary Entry: BCBS, 5/16/2003 Sinking Fast...

The patient of the day–58, male, educated, high functioning, no history of MH or TX (treatment), goes into his garage, puts noose around his neck and stands on a stool–someone walks in on him...ends up in a psych hospital. Sometimes, I wish that was me...Greg is looking for a replacement in Quality Improvement. I would be good at this...Nina tells me to apply. I'm so miserable–David tells me I made a huge mistake moving to BCBS....

For a short time before I left the Aetna Team, I contemplated starting a newsletter for care managers. When the rules of the company would not permit a newsletter in which it did not control the content, I thought I would start a small, private venture so that I could write, manage and print it independently. Then, under the darkness of night, I would deliver my *Care Manager's Advocate* to neighboring coffee houses, delis and restaurants surrounding managed care offices. Unfortunately, this fantasy remained in my imagination...and my diary.

The Care Manager's Advocate
July 2002

A company that respects its employees has productive employees. Are you respected at Magellan? Send in your anonymous comments. Magellan is banking on care managers' "buy in" for the company's future. Have you?

Fantasy Letter from Corporate:

"My Most Valued Care Managers,

I wish to thank you all for your dedicated, albeit dogged loyalty and diligence over the last year and a half. You have suffered through the previous administration's reckless decision to impose the Time Tracking System which was subsequently found to be invalid. You have bravely endured through several layoff episodes and a newer and harsher administration. And, adding insult to injury, we also discovered that not all centers were using it. In the end you have never received an apology for this: I am truly sorry this happened to you. Also during this time, you lost a beloved president, heard about the company's bankruptcy and upcoming reorganization, anxiously witnessed two layoff episodes and wearily watched the parking spaces dwindle away while your workload increased. And now? Now you are being asked to tighten you belts for the lean times and hold on to your hat for the world wind of changes to come. This means taking more calls, more cases, more certs, having more training, cross training, meetings, and instructions about more details. Some of you are asking yourselves: "Does anyone care about retaining care managers around here?" We value you, we need you, we celebrate you."

Tired of the retraining and the chaos created from it, care managers knew "managed" care had become so badly mismanaged and that we had become puppets. Having been told that "corporate" wanted us to cross train so that we could be moved as needed, morale was low, turnover high. Yet I was determined to hold on to this job for the income, which I doubted I could get elsewhere, and because of the unpleasant notion of job hunting at age 52. Many of my colleagues felt the same way. Every monthly meeting brought new announcements of changes. Further, we were blamed for not making the new plans work! Helplessness and hopelessness loomed above us.

The Care Manager's Advocate

October 2002

10/14/2002

CAREMANAGER FLIPS OFF TIMETRACKING
FOR "REAL" CAREMANAGEMENT

IT'S 4:05 ON FRIDAY AFTERNOON. CM IS FINISHING OFF LAST
CONCURRENT REVIEW. NEXT WILL BE CLEANUP OF CENSUS
THEN IT WILL BE 4:30, TIME TO GO HOME. THERE'S AN IN-
COMING CALL- "DON'T ANSWER IT, IT'S PROBABLY NOTHING
IMPORTANT" BUT THE OTHER VOICE WINS—"IT MIGHT BE
SOMETHING IMPORTANT"— ON VM: UR AT FACILITY TELLING
ME PT "V" DID NOT D/C AS WE DISCUSSED EARLIER.
THOUGHTS RACING THRU CM'S MIND: CERT THE WEEKEND?
GET CLINICAL? IS UR STILL THERE? PA? NOW? WEEKEND?
PT IS MANIPULATIVE, NOT REALLY A RISK—WILL WEEKEND
DOCS KNOW THIS CASE, THIS PT? I'VE GOT TO TALK TO MD.
WHO'S STILL HERE? CAN I DO IT THIS LATE? WHERE'S NINA?
CM JUMPS TO HER FEET, SEES NINA'S DOOR OPENED. RUNS
TO CONSULT, NINA AGREES GO AHEAD AND PA, DR REDDY
STILL HERE. CM RACES TO DR REDDY'S OFFICE — IT'S 4: 30.
YES, DR REDDY CAN DO IT –MUST BE RIGHT AWAY . CM RACES
BACK TO PREPARE PA, TAKES 20 MIN—.
ANOTHER CM YELLS OUT: "WAYNETTE WANTS TO KNOW IF
ANYONE ELSE HAS A PA", CM YELLS BACK: "TELL HER YES,
I DO, I DO".   CM RACING TO GET ALL NOTES TO WAYNETTE.
CM CALLS WAYNETTE TELLING HER DR REDDY IS READY RIGHT
NOW TO DO PA, LETS GET IT TO HIM, ASAP , IT'S
5 TO 5.   WAYNETTE INFORMING ME THAT DR POLE NOT
AVAILABLE AFTER 4 PM AND REQUIRES 24 HOUR NOTICE FOR
PA. CM ASKING WAYNETTE TO CALL MAIN NUMBER AND HAVE
HER PAGED AT HOSP OR CALL TONI. CM RUSHES BACK TO
NINA'S OFFICE ASKING "WHAT ABOUT A PAPER REVIEW SINCE
DR POLE NOT AVAILABLE?" NINA SAYS, "WHY NOT?" THIS IS
OK.   BUT DR REDDY THINKS AETNA WILL AUTOMATICALLY
OVERTURN SUCH A REVIEW. NINA SAYING "NO". DR REDDY
STARTS TO HUNT DOWN DR POLE... AND HE FINDS HER ON A
BACK LINE.   BUT HE DOES NOT HAVE NOTES YET. IN THE
MEANTIME, CM ATTEMPTING TO FINISH ALL NOTES, AUTHS,
CENSUS CLEANUP— CM BEGINS TO CLOSE DOWN, E-MAIL,
AMSW, ETC AND IS ABOUT TO LOG OUT. DR REDDY ASKS CM

FOR NOTES SINCE HE NEEDS THEM RIGHT AWAY TO DISCUSS
WITH DR POLE. IT IS NOW 5:30. CM PULLS UP AMSW, COPIES
NOTES AND E-MAILS TO DR REDDY. DR REDDY COMPLETES
REVIEW, DENIES FURTHER STAY. BOTH DOCS AGREE PT DOES
NOT MEET MNC FOR CONT STAY IN INPT LOC. CM LOGGED OUT
AT 5:50PM.

THERE WAS NO TIME FOR TIME TRACKING IN THIS 2 HR AND 45
MIN DRAMA. IF CM HAD BEEN USING TIME TRACKING IT
WOULD INDEED HAVE IMPEDED THE CM'S ABILITY TO USE
GOOD JUDGEMENT AND RESPOND IMMEDIATELY.
CM SAVED MAGELLAN 3 DAYS OF INPT CERT BY COORDINAT-
ING ALL PARTIES TOWARD THE BEST DECISION FOR
THIS CASE. YET BY TIME TRACKING STANDARDS, CM 'S
PERFORMANCE WENT DOWN SIGNIFICANTLY.

CM WORKED AN HOUR AND 20 MINUTES OVER TIME, SAVED
THE COMPANY MONEY AND HELPED TO GATHER INFO ABOUT A
PT THAT COULD INFLUENCE HIS FUTURE RELATIONSHIP WITH
AETNA. BUT CM'S PERFORMANCE IS VERY POOR FOR THIS
DAY ACCORDING TO TIME TRACKING.

Bureaucratic bloat meets rancid soup...

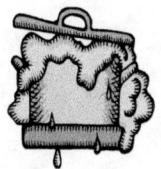

PART II Chap 4

BAD PR:

MISINFORMATION ABOUT MENTAL ILLNESS

Why this is important and someone slap that journalist

Feb 23, 2005, Fox News Channel anchor interviews journalist in the field who just finished her report about yet another teacher who sexually perpetrated one of her students:

> <u>Anchor:</u> "What about this, Janet, this kind of incident to be on the rise...? Is there any way we can be preventing this ...some kind of screening we can do to weed out these kinds of people from being exposed to our children?"
>
> <u>Reporter:</u> "Well, not really, Allen, I mean, what are you going to do? You can't very well ask these people if they have plans to molest a child....".
>
> (Report, Fox News Channel, 2005)

And so it goes; two journalists asking each other dumb questions instead of doing the footwork necessary to uncover the truth and reporting that. In the end, the sound bite makes the news instead of the actual facts in the story.

In a typical piece written about the Columbine shootings, the journalist is describing the "young man" as a "quiet, shy.......". But as the story unfolds the facts surface that each of the perpetrators of this horrendous crime had a tell-tale history of chaotic or broken families and anti social behaviors. The author calls these cases "The Happy Family" syndrome. For some reason, reporters love to have us believe that aberrations of humanity occur even in the "happy family". In fact, this implies that parents are helpless and maybe even useless. Whereas parents do not have total control over their children's' behaviors and choices, they certainly have a lot more influence than the "victim" bunch would have us believe.

"Happy Family"? Show me the messed up kid and I will show you the messed up family! Unless one accepts the "bad seed" theory, children are basically formed by their families. Ask around, interview the teacher, investigate the previous teacher or the principal of his school. Ask about previous trouble with local authorities. When was the last time the parents went into their garage? Hello? Who is supervising the adolescent? Where are the parents? Who are the parents? You went to school for this *journalism* ?

Binghamton, NY, Friday, April 3rd, 2009:

The Hobbs News Sun blasts this headline:

"Rampage 'was not a surprise'".

And then this:

"It remains unclear exactly why the Vietnamese immigrant strapped on a bullet proof vest, barged in on a citizenship class and killed 13 people and himself...".

The article goes on to name a number of possible precipitants to this heinous act from being made fun of, loss of job and anger at America. Though it was noted that his friends reported that the gunman felt anger at America for years, none talked about his childhood, where it all starts. Their research goes as far back as his twenties when he moved from Vietnam to America and became a citizen. He lived in several states, had several jobs, one he quit and another he was fired from. He was unemployed but taking classes to improve his English. But despite the obvious opportunities that benefited this madman in this country, the focus is on the *awful American economic situation.* This journalist, like so many others would benefit from Mental Health 101, information that should be out there for anyone who follows the human condition and events. Lack of acknowledgment of the effects of this criminal's family history is a significant shortcoming among our citizenry.

The media is often clueless assisted by journalists who misrepresent serious mental disorders without research or investigation.. Now don't get me wrong here; I am not suggesting that journalists need to become mental health professionals. But some degree of common sense should enter the minds of these folks regarding human behavior. Kids, and people in general do not behave erratically in a vacuum: something always precedes an unusual incident. The precipitant is usually years and years and years of serious neglect, maltreatment, and bad genes. I am reminded of a preteen I once worked with. When I asked him how he came to the psychiatric facility, he stated: "My mother drove me".   It's this type of juvenile mentality that we see exhibited by our journalists when they report in short time capsule style about the incidences that they "cover". Get the background!

Diary Entry: BCBS, 5/28/03 The New Guy...

Was confused and overwhelmed at work again today.. Discovered I have been given the bottom of the barrel facilities—no wonder they're always going PA (aka. Peer Review) and I'm chasing them for discharge plans. This team is truly the "ghetto" as one of my fellow care managers likes to call it. They see me struggling but pay no attention to me—there is nothing but sarcasm and bathroom jokes among them...they are sort of immature, mean even.

But I know they have low self esteem here—they are expected to just authorize everything without question, without analysis or consultation... like robots. Their jobs are meaningless... But wait; here comes the new CM, being treated with kid gloves....he's got a personal trainer sitting on his lap eight hours a day...not like the flimsy treatment I got. He's someone's favorite...So what am I–chopped liver???? Four weeks on Prozac and no improvement....

Another media "culprit" is Hollywood. Movies and television shows portraying the mentally ill tend to elaborate on the most bizarre elements of the condition. Only recently have producers considered movies that accurately tell the story of the mentally ill. "A Beautiful Mind" was one such movie, and this author's hope is that more worthy films on this topic will follow. In the meantime, there is non-stop misinformation coming to us via our entertainment industry. Portrayals of mental illness are designed to capture our attention or sway us this way or that, or just shock us: mental issues are a perfect food for our unlimited imaginations and craving for the bizarre. The movie "Sybil" comes to mind. We are captivated by cases of young mothers who drown their children in a bathtub or depraved killers who bind and rape women. Some of the accused are, or claim to be, mentally ill. This becomes the foundation of our "education" about mental illness. We learn about depression from talk show hosts and women's magazines and consider ourselves enlightened. We say things like: "Well, everyone experiences depression at some time in their lives", and come to believe that maybe depression can make you *kill* people, or maybe all those psychiatrist types are really quacks because depression *doesn't* make you *kill* people. We are obsessed with the notion of *depression,* abusing and misusing the definition, even taking sides for and against the its existence. But here is the actual diagnoses for Major Depressive Disorder which begins with the diagnosis of an "episode" of depression:

"A. Five or more of the following symptoms have been present during the same two week period and represent a change from previous functioning: at least one of the symptoms is either 1. Depressed mood or, 2. loss of interest or pleasure.

Note: does not include symptoms that are clearly due to a general medical condition, or mood-incongruent delusions or hallucinations.

1. Depressed mood most of the day, as indicated by either subjective report or observation by others

2. Markedly diminished interest or pleasure in all or almost all activities most of the day, nearly every day as indicated by either subjective account or observation made by others

3. Significant weight loss when not dieting or weight gain (more than 5% of body weight in a month), or decrease or increase of appetite nearly every day.

4. Insomnia or hyper-somnia nearly every day

5. Psychomotor agitation or retardation nearly every day (observable by others not just subjective feelings or restlessness or being slowed down)

6. Fatigue or loss of energy nearly every day

7. Feelings of worthlessness or excessive or inappropriate guilt (which may be delusional) nearly every day (not just self-reproach or guilt about being sick).

8. Diminished ability to think or concentrate, or indecisiveness, nearly every day (either by subjective account or as observed by others)

9. *Recurrent thoughts of death (not just fear of dying), recurrent suicidal ideation without a specific plan, or a suicide attempt, or a specific plan for committing suicide.*

B.   The symptoms are not part of a "mixed" episode

C.   The symptoms cause clinically significant distress, or impairment in social, occupational, or other important areas of functioning.

D.   The symptoms are not due to a direct physiological effects of a substance or medical condition (such as hypothyroidism)

E.   The symptoms are not due to bereavement (loss of loved one) or symptoms persist for longer than two months or are characterized by marked function impairment, morbid preoccupation with worthlessness, suicidal ideation, psychotic symptoms, or psychomotor retardation."

(DSM, 2004, pp 739-740)

The above formal description of one episode (incident) of Major Depressive Disorder drives home the point that a clinical condition is much more extensive than just feeling "down" for a few days, as it is often believed by the general public. So what is the solution to our ignorance? Advocacy on the part of the mental health community, more public relations campaigns, more emphasis on mental health in the schools, and better trained journalists, perhaps?

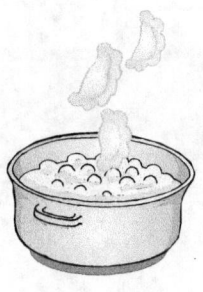

PART III

SUFFER THE CHILDREN

We have become a people comfortable with the notion that government owes us many services. This applies to behavioral health care as well. Put in general terms, fewer people are willing to accept responsibility for their own problems. Still, even fewer people think they should pay to fix their own problems. As if it were not enough that the MBHO system contributes to the rise of health care costs through mismanagement, damaged care enables the continuation of the "entitlement mentality" Preying on the under informed and vulnerable of our citizenry it opens loopholes for the greedy and irresponsible.

In this section, the author discusses the loose parameters which define mental illness and how the lines blur to accommodate social ills. This impacts our children who are entered into the system by their uninformed and often irresponsible parents. Make no mistake about it, attitudes and values are inculcated at a very young age through role modeling of the adults around the child. Finally, we will look at Medicaid which has expanded to encompasses every excuse to freeload imaginable to human kind.

Not surprisingly, this coincides with the way our country is headed; nearly half of the current population receives some type of subsidy.

Diary Entry: BCBS, 6/22/09,

Still crying about the "PA talk" with Desi and Lucy... I should have reminded them that all my PAs are upheld! Doesn't that count?! I hate myself, I can't seem to hold my own, defend myself, but I can't leave. God put me here for a reason—not to be other than myself—but to be who I am, to have an impact, no? I did this to myself without praying about it... I moved from Aetna to BCBS... Aetna, where my work was known, where attempts to improve things were honored—but wait! I was not respected there either! I was called a traitor by Nina for wanting to leave the team.. leave the never-ending screens, the three day hospital stays, the Time Tracking torture...

I guess today got me because I went into action on a case and discovered how uninformed the supervisors and team members are on this team... And these are the people who are supposed to evaluate me??? Desi and Lucy don't want to discuss how all my PAs are <u>upholds</u>. So Maryanna is a assistant supervisor and Scott is a QI expert and I am an inadequate CM! Oh, holy God, are you trying to tell me I can't fight city hall? Or am I supposed to be opening people's eyes.... I don't have the strength but I don't want to be a *quitter;* then Lucy and Desi win....

PART III CHAP 1

UNDEFINED SERVICES/DUBIOUS RECIPIENTS

Mental Illness or Social Ills?

Question: What do behavioral problems in children and teens have in common with recurring drunks?

Here it is: They are not mentally ill; they cannot benefit from services for the mentally ill; they are socially ill and they are a drain on the MBHO system and the tax payers; they are forever succeeding at ripping off and manipulating same system. Unfortunately, some psychiatrists and mental health professionals may be assisting them with the assignment of embellished diagnoses and the promise of unrealistic results to line their own pockets   What about all these populations which continue to drain on the services for the mentally ill? There are facilities and providers that are ethical and will not admit these clients to services for which they are not appropriate.   But the industry is very creative and comes up with programs and services to meet the needs of all sorts of folks.   Don't want to go to jail? How about a rehab center? Don't want your teenager to be suspended?   Get him a diagnosis of Major Depression and ADHD and a script for Zoloft and Ritalin and hook him up with a few therapy sessions. Fall off the wagon again? Just slink away to that Sunrise Ranch out in the woods for a nice long twenty eight days of drying out rest. Your neighborly taxpayer, I mean HMO/PPO will pay for that for you! We watch in dismay as our premiums rise...

Friends, this is another racket. Your money and mine is being sucked into it by the managed behavioral health care bureaucracy, their supporters, and some unsavory practitioners and facilities. Local and federal government programs for all the sorry individuals who cannot pay for healthcare and don't fit under the mental health umbrella are also to blame. Face it: people are being "treated" for free on your tax dime for illnesses they don't have! This, while the authentically mentally ill often go misunderstood and untreated.

Another population impacting health care services are teen parents who pass their young children off to aging grandparents who tend to be derelict in the supervision department. This family "model" is prevalent in some cultures where one can also find the highest incidence of teen and out of wedlock births. the highest incidence of poverty, unemployment, drug use, criminal activity and school dropout rates. Chaos prevails throughout their generations and they may be on publicly funded plans or uninsured. While "profiling" groups of people who harbor most of the social ills of society is not exactly politically correct, our denial prevents us from focusing true corrective action, not just money, in their direction. Remember? Teach them to fish?

Between the inefficient managed care system, the treatment of social ills, the pretend patients and irresponsible assignment of mental illness diagnoses, and government interference in the healthcare industry, one should not be surprised that health care costs are rising out of control.

Contributing to Delinquency

Now of all members of our population who would readers think is better equipped to know and understand human nature than the mental health practitioner? One would think! While most of us who choose this field are benevolent types who want to save or cure people, to ease their pain, to remove the obstacles that impede the normal functioning of life. but often there are selfish motives that belie these longings. Some may want to preserve a personal image or ego, some may have unresolved needs of their own that were never met, and still others just feel good when others feel bad! Who can discern among them? This is a problem for the mental health professional community. Since impaired judgment is common among many recipients of mental health services and ignorance is common among many of the socially ill, it is difficult to choose the appropriate provider or service. In addition, many well meaning but self ordained "healers" try to "treat" folks who may require professional services. One such example is the unlicensed minister who attends to an individual with an undiagnosed mental illness and unwittingly believes the issue to be a spiritual one. Another example is the recovering alcoholics who become drug and alcohol counselors and assume this prepares them to treat depression and bipolar disorders as well.

This author teaches Master's level counseling students who are studying for a degree and/ or licensure to do this type of work. My experience has been that, as a whole, this population does authentically seek to help people and to gain the proper credentials to do so. But the environments they will work in may prevent them from doing so. An example of this would be the psychiatric hospital which admits the "dubious patients" in order to drain their insurance, or skimps on the services to a seriously mentally ill patient to enlarge their profits. Another example is the clinic which must follow so many state and insurance regulations that treatment is hampered. Still another example would be the private practice mental health provider who finds it necessary to "recruit patients" or stretch out their treatment services to keep the business afloat. And the author is familiar with some public schools who give their counselor the role of disciplining children in addition to counseling them. This particular example is a dire situation in our schools today. At a crucial time in a child's life when a serious emotional issue should be addressed, the child is instead "treated" for his misbehavior! Surely if I were a child I would not disclose anything of significance to these *counselors!*

These types of practices lead to a watering down of the definition of the mentally ill and give support to the "takers" who also benefit from receiving unneeded services. Before we know it, an industry exists which creates and encourages "patients" to visit counselors who would otherwise have to function without crutches and excuses like the rest of us!

Medical Necessity Criteria– Why isn't this clear to everyone?

This author can produce multiple and varied charts and cheat sheets of the definitions of Medical Necessity Criteria (MNC discussed earlier in this book). Yet MNC is used to determine whether or not services will be covered by the MBHO. Here is an area that really needs standardization! Cigna likes to call its MNC manual "Level of Care Guidelines" (6/16/03). This booklet features a father holding his two small children and they are all smiling and content looking. Next comes the bad news:

"In considering the appropriateness of any level of

care, the five basic elements of Medical Necessity should be met:

1. A diagnosis as defined by standard diagnostic nomenclatures (DSM—Diagnostic & Statistical Manual which lists and defines every mental disorder), and an individualized treatment plan appropriate for the participant's illness or condition.

2. A reasonable expectation that the participant's illness, condition, or level of functioning will improve through treatment known to be effective for the participant's illness.

3. Consistent in type, frequency and duration of treatment with scientifically based guidelines as determined by medical research and/or expert consensus clinical decisions

4. It is the most appropriate and cost-effective level of care that can safely be provided for the participant's immediate condition and rendered in the least intensive setting.

5. Required for purposes other than avoidance of incarceration, comfort and   convenience of the patient or his/her family, or his/her treating practitioner." (Level of Care Guidelines, Cigna, 2003)

One rather renowned psychiatric facility this author worked

for had an entire unit dedicated to the treatment of multiple personality disorder. MPD, now known as DID or Dissociative Identity Disorder is a very rare condition in which the personality splits into two or more separate and distinct personalities in order to escape from a traumatic experience or the memory of one. Many people think this is easy to fake and indeed they attempt to present as DID for whatever reason. But trained psychiatrists and mental health professionals can, for the most part, ascertain who the phonies are. For one thing, memory loss and lack of knowledge of other identities or what they do is often a symptom in the early stages of this disorder. Patients came from all over the country to be in this program. The author would not venture to guess what percentage of this population was not appropriate for inpatient care at a psychiatric hospital, but my experience was that if the patient claimed to be suicidal then that was enough to get in and stay in. One would be surprised how many individuals would love to spend a couple of weeks or more at a psychiatric facility...

The author's point is this: human beings tend not to care what services cost when they are not paying for them and the fact is that all of us pay for it. This is how the entitlement mentality grows. Entitlement then breeds further demand for more free services. But wait, readers may ask, why shouldn't those of us who pay insurance premiums and co pays receive whatever services we desire or require?   The answer is this: your premiums and co pays do not cover all the services you desire or require!   The one size fits all package of premiums and co pays means that all of us will at some time pay more and use less, and others of us at some time will pay less than the cost of the services we receive. My favorite analogy is the grading system in a typical classroom. In a nutshell, work very hard and earn an A, work less and earn a B or a C, work as little as possible and earn a D, do not work at all and earn an F. This bears no resemblance to the current damaged care system. Instead, we follow an inequitable system wherein every class member gets a C no matter how much or how little each works! Translation: We do not pay for what we think we deserve, but some other healthy person is probably paying for us...

In summary, managed care is just as guilty as Medicaid in creating an entitlement mentality among American citizens. This is miles away from our founding fathers' vision of individual responsibility, self determination and participation in a consumer driven economy. As a matter of fact, it resembles socialism. Sadly, the takers and their cohorts who support the redistribution of wealth and health are under the impression that getting something for nothing is a good thing. It puzzles and disturbs this author that the Soup Pot proponents cannot see the dastardly consequences .

Entitlement Mentality

We hear a lot lately about our culture becoming one with an "entitlement mentality".

As I understand it, this is when a segment or more of the population comes to believe that their government owes them many free services, goods and/ or financial compensation. This mentality develops when their government gives special populations these awards. Those receiving the awards come to expect them and want even more, while those who do not receive them come to feel jealous and find ways to be "eligible" for same awards. Now, once this becomes easier to do, the practical among us start to wonder if it is "worth it" to continue to work hard to gain goods, services and compensation when they can be gotten from the 'gift horse', the government. So the next level of income earners drop out of the work force to join their fellow "takers". None of these folks stop to ask the question: "Who is paying for all of us to live like free spirits?" Why it is the rest of us of course! This leads to low morale and motivation to excel. The more the rest of us make, the higher our taxes go and the more of the "takers" we have to support! For whom does this course of events not make sense? Those without knowledge or understanding of human nature, that is who.

Diary Entry: BCBS, 6/5/03 More of the Same...

Ok, I will admit it–I tried to set them up. Desi and Lucy had another pow-wow with me ...I guess they are accumulating "documentation" about what a terrible CM I am... These meeting are crushing me... I am acting dumb: How exactly can I figure out when to automatically authorize Partial Hospitalization and when to loosely interpret medical necessity criteria and how to write it up in the notes for the case? I hoped I could get them to say "Fix the notes, falsify the documentation! But my plan backfired–proof that I am not very good at playing games... Now they want me to bring my cases to them before I send it to PA.... Guess what? –they are never around to go to! So I sit and wait while cases pile, letters are not going out in a timely manner, my phone is ringing off the hook---- Again I walked out of Desi's office with my tail between my legs...

PART III CHAP 2

"NOT MY CHILD!"

News Flash: Parents who do not take full responsibility for their children and their children's well being tend to raise children who also don't take responsibility for their actions. And when families are fractured and "blended" and displaced, children rebel by developing dysfunctional behaviors. In other words, IT'S THE FAMILY STUPID!!!!! Along these same lines my grandmother would say, "The apple does not fall far from the tree". Teaching children to be victims of their world is the antithesis of the messages which built the American culture and dream. It also backfires on parents when children refuse to follow the family rules, talk back and are generally oppositional or even threatening. The author has spoken with countless parents through the MBHO system as a care manager, mostly when they were desperate. But the cast has been dyed and desperate measures are often indicated. Here's an important question that should be part of any Family History Questionnaire:

Where were YOU when your child was birth to five years of age, the most critical developmental years?

I posed this question to a parent policyholder who was seeking an RTC camp, I mean, "treatment center" for her sixteen year old son who had stolen the family car, wrecked it, received two DUIs and been suspended from school for trafficking in marijuana and cocaine on school property. This was not meant to be a rhetorical question; the author understands and appreciates the impact of the family environment in the early years and relies heavily on this information. The parent was unable to answer the question because she was the boy's second step mother. She didn't really know the adolescent's history. She had not considered that by marrying the boy's biological father, she may become responsible for the teenager. Say what?! The media and Hollywood have conditioned this generation of parents to believe that multiple partnering and multiple parenting is acceptable and that child rearing just happens regardless of parents' actions. In addition, not only is it unacceptable to discourage single parenting but it is to be glorified. The author is not stating anything new here: the family unit has undergone devastating changes for our youngsters.

Diary Entry: BCBS, 6/30/2009,

Slap in the face...

Today I wanted to run screaming from that place... I am on the After Hours line, it's the end of the day for everyone else and I am supposed to handle the phone alone for one hour before I can go home... This is the Queue, the unpredictable line... The ghetto CMs are huddling in the back of the row with Witch Lucy whispering and telling bathroom jokes, tearing other teams apart and generally acting like adolescents... Now here comes a call from an irate parent wanting to know why her son's case was denied... I'm tired, I'm down and out, disgusted, overwhelmed and listening while the mother shouts at me... I motion to Lucy, the, ah, assistant supervisor, to come and help me... I'm desperate, feeling helpless. Lucy makes a joke with the rest of the ghetto residents and glares at me–I'm in tears–and walks up to my desk smirking–"You handle it! I'm off the clock!"

Banished to the RTC: "Take my kid, please!"

Enter the RTC. Residential Treatment Centers or programs offer a secluded second residence to children and adolescents who are "out of control" per their parents or who have just plain been dumped. They administer "treatment" in the form of extended counseling and activities which build self esteem, trust and self awareness. They make a killing off the fears and frustrations of battle fatigued parents who do not know how to regain control of their offspring. After the initial denial that the family has anything whatever to do with Jeffrey's bizarre behaviors, parents beg professionals to "fix" their kids. Their calls pour in to the MBHO and Intake personnel who can barely contain their weeping and demanding pleas for us to DO SOMETHING! Typical calls include but are not limited to the following:

1. Jeffrey has found a gun and is threatening his parents

2. Julie has cut her wrists and we are on the way to the ER

3. Joshua has written a paper about his bomb invention

4. Julio hit his principal at school.

5. Jessica is refusing to eat, go to school, come out of her room

6. Jamie overdosed on heroin, cocaine, whatever drug of choice

But the behavior is not recent; it does not exist in a vacuum. It has been going on "ever since we moved", "ever since the divorce", "ever since Uncle Frank moved in", or whatever. In the minds of some clueless parents it started "last week" when the child client was given an unappealing rule to follow. The author is reminded of the parent who explained that her teenage daughter *just started* acting out after visiting her father in jail who molested her when she was five. Does this have anything to do with the child's unhealed wounds from the sexual abuse itself? Is it apathy or ignorance that drives the clueless parent?

And the remedies tried have all failed, or perhaps the police have entered the picture, or some other consequences have resulted. Substance abuse is usually a component. And bad parenting is *always* a component unless there is an underlying medical condition. But mental health professionals do not want to appear as if they are "passing judgment". It's not politically correct. Dare I say these ugly next words? It serves many professionals well to have consumers believe that the problem is much more *esoteric* and can be "cured" only by the specialists. There, I have said it. Not only is the family the *precipitant* of the problem, but it started in the earliest years of the child's life. Selfish parents opt for divorce before considering the effects on their children. Selfish single parents opt to bring home multiple partners before considering their children. Unfit parents bring more fatherless children into the world. Absentee fathers and mothers abandon their offspring or engage in substance abuse and other risky behaviors. Bad parents happen...

I regret that a mental illness diagnosis is easy to come by if you are a persistent parent. There are plenty of appropriate labels for kids who are out of control such as "Oppositional

Defiant Disorder", "Pervasive Developmental Disorder", "Reactive Attachment Disorder", "ADHD", and my favorite, "Intermittent Explosive Disorder". There are claims that some of these disorders are neurological in nature and even hereditary. The author is not insinuating that the disorders don't exist; only that they are sometimes overused and their treatment outcomes are dubious. Parents have every right to look into these maladies if they believe their child has the stated symptoms. And it behooves parents to take the recommendations of their mental health providers ---after checking them out thoroughly and getting a second opinion if necessary.

But overused labels encourage mentalities that release the child or adolescent from responsibility, and burden our system with demands for more "services". And more *free* services! If asked pointedly, the ethical psychiatrist will inform parents that there is *no difinitive treatment* nor *medicine* for ODD or IED or even ADHD (with the exception of some medications that can alleviate some symptoms). In addition, many of the medications used for these conditions have life changing side effects. And in fact, the "patient" has a *behavioral problem* and *not* a mental illness. Sometimes, the over inflated diagnosis is used to keep the child out of jail and get him or her into rehab. As a care manager this author encountered cases of burned out parents who, needing a "break" from their unruly teenagers, attempted to exaggerate the child's symptoms to get them into a rehab center. Then there are the cases of children who are faced with school suspension for their behaviors. Cases of enabling parents, ineffective parents, multiple step parents, blended family syndrome issues– all of these crowd into the psychiatrist's office and consider themselves candidates for mental health services. Are they? The author is in favor of family counseling and serious changes to the family system first, while pursuing a more accurate diagnosis for the minor patient. When parents are unwilling to change to help their children get well, hear this all providers: *nothing will work*. This is the challenge of changing children's lives and futures that mental health providers face, and a difficult one to accept. Rather than trying to fix the broken child from the uncooperative and dysfunctional family, more focus should be placed on preventive care such as parenting classes. (The author might consider an education and *licensing* program for new parents). As long as our citizens–even the worst citizens among us- have an unlimited "right" to have children, there will be a population of abused, neglected and discarded children. This of course, is a very controversial topic...

Diary Entry: BCBS, 7/6/09, While Desi is away...

David being on vacation has brought the worst out in Lucy.

I think she's threatened by me because I know so much more than she does. I think my team mates are to.. Why don't these flashes of wisdom comfort me when I feel worthless, ignored and incompetent? We get into a conflict over a case...she tells me I am not doing my job...What will Desi say when he returns from vacation? Is this the end of the line for me? I go to the HR person to report I am being harassed-bad move! She toes the company line... I'm scared and alone-no one is going to investigate what really goes on the BS Team—it's BS! Everything is authorized regardless of criteria, partial is given away, there are "unspoken rules", uninformed and incompetent supervisors, cm s who are demoralized and unmotivated... doctors who don't take their jobs seriously—just do whatever is expected of them... If I quit, then I am the one who loses...I'm out there hitting the pavement with a mortgage to pay by myself....when I am not the one who is corrupt! God, I can hear Job crying to you... Quit? Stay and make a point? Be a whistle blower? Does anyone but me care???

Partial Day = Partial Solution

Another prefabricated program concocted by this industry is the "day program", also known as the "partial hospitalization program", or the "partial day program". What a dilemma this poses for the parent. The notion of dumping a child in an RTC or a psychiatric hospital overnight may seem scary, but how about an all day long program that even includes school? It sounds like the perfect compromise. The facility staff or the house psychiatrist (if available) presents an appealing package: two process groups per day, lunch, two breaks, individual therapy, family therapy, physical therapy, perhaps some musical or art therapy, and "trust building" activities and even school! What a deal! Now, some discrepancies usually exist with the admission criteria for these programs. The program accepts children and adolescents if they claim to have suicidal thoughts, known as "passive suicidality", *or children of parents who are willing to pay out of pocket.* The managed care company will cover this only if the child patient is actually suicidal with plan and intent. Though this is very different from actually demonstrating suicidality, as in a suicide attempt, it requires more than just a statement by the child that he/she has "suicidal thoughts". Suffice it to say, the definitions for suicidality and passive suicidality are a matter of continued controversy among mental health professionals and serious liability for managed care companies and providers. How much more complex this issue is for children and adolescents. At BCBS this CM was instructed to "step down" every RTC patient to Partial Program with the same facility. The ruckus that followed when this automatic rule was challenged provides another indictment of managed care. The author had come to understand the MNC (medical necessity criteria in Dictionary,

Part II) to mean that the patient was still suicidal. But after several weeks in a full time RTC this condition had already been addressed. In fact, Discharge Criteria demanded that suicidality be resolved prior to discharge. Why then are we stepping the patient down to a partial program for hundreds of dollars per day for an additional two weeks or more when this is presumably reserved for those who are suicidal? The powers that were did not like this kind of questioning ...

And, according to the Medical Necessity manual,

> "This level of care (partial day) should not be confused with the long-term sub acute "day programs" where the focus is more on social rehabilitation and maintenance of participants with severe and persistent mental illness. This level of care should not be considered as an alternative for participants where the school system has not provided the alternative academic setting."
> (CBH Level of Care Guidelines ,2003)

But it is exactly these blurred lines that make these standards impotent. Partial hospitalization often morphs into the day program where children and teens may languish indefinitely. This is made possible because 1. There is a contract between the provider facility and the managed care company which guarantees them mutual profit, and, 2. There are doctors on the managed care staff who may also work as consultant, board member or even director of that very same provider facility! Now some readers may think this type of incestuous relationship actually increases treatment for children. These readers would be correct! So is the goal increased treatment or quality treatment? In the long run, there are less dollars for the rest of the population which may have more needs. The least ill are paying for the most ill. Taxes increase and premiums rise.

There is increased treatment under these weak MNC and blurred Level of Care Guidelines, given the games between the providers and managed care. Litigation is a constant and real threat. And most of it is waste or overkill and causes taxpayers' premiums to rise! Torte reform is so needed. So while the clients believe they are entitled to this type of service and grateful that their doctor, managed care company and the facility provider are all recommending it, they are clueless that they will "pay" for it in the large scheme of things. In fact, this is why no one has blown the whistle on the whole managed care paradigm in its current form. It appears on the surface as if everyone wins, when in fact, only managed care and providers win. In addition, as mentioned earlier, children and teens are turned into victims, their parents seeking labels and services for them for the remainder of their underage lives. Defraying responsibility for the child's plight, and avoiding the hard work of change within the family through family counseling sells well with desperate and guilt ridden parents. So, what is it like inside a psychiatric facility? Not fun for a 4 or 14 year old!

Suicidality and Children

Mental Health professionals have heard these statements from child clients perhaps just slightly more than parents have:

"I HATE YOU! I'M GOING TO KILL YOU!"

"I HATE MYSELF! I'M GOING TO KILL MYSELF!"

What we really want to know is: When is it really a risk? The CDC reports that suicide is the third leading cause of death among 15-24 year olds. (Suicide, Facts At a Glance, 2007). I bring this up in this section because there are serious risks and concerns for our children–even those without a legitimate diagnosis of major depressive disorder. While we most certainly want the MBHO to cover this treatment, I am not so sure they are equipped to assess the risks in the current environment of Queue calls, harried care managers and bullying supervisors. My recommendation here is face to face evaluation of the child or adolescent by a well chosen licensed professional.

One of my favorite authors on the subject of suicidality and how it is assessed is M. David Rudd, Ph.D., ABPP. In one of his workshops, *Lives and Liability: Suicide Risk Assessment, Clinical Management and Documentation*, (2004), Dr. Rudd suggests that suicidal thoughts be examined carefully. For example, the child or adolescent should be asked how often these thoughts occur and under what circumstances. Determine whether the thoughts have increased, decreased or remain constant. What kinds of statements are being used? For example: "I wish I were dead" or "I would be better off dead" or "I wish I was never born" are passive statements and considered less risky than say, suicidality "with a plan". The interviewer should make an effort to find out about the child or adolescent's attitude toward life and death and the history of plans or attempts. Another question asks "What is the means by which the suicide will take place?", and another, "How available is the means?" Still another asks, "What are the barriers to committing suicide?" or "What has prevented you from doing it so far?" Another important consideration is how impulsive the child or adolescent is. Know the demographics of risk; suicide is generally prevalent among males, forty-five years and up who live alone and are unemployed or retired. But teens hold the second highest risk rates.

Early or recent life losses, health problems, mental health issues, irritability, helplessness are all risk factors for suicide. The risks are greater when under the influence of alcohol or substances, and when there is a family history of suicide.

While anyone can proclaim suicidal thought, there is the matter of intent. While anyone can feel suicidal at a given time, there is the matter of plan and means. One five year old told his parents he wanted to kill himself by dunking his head in the bathtub. What does a parent or mental health professional make of that? Research in child development informs us that children do not even *understand* death prior to age ten. Whatever the consequences, children's television portrays characters that come back to life shortly after "dying". Some of this is actually quite funny to them.

Does the MBHO have a better handle on cases of child or teen suicidality than the rest of the mental health community? I doubt it. But the assessment of risk should certainly be carried out by a trained professional who is not under undue time constraints, computer anxieties, and template exhaustion! Perhaps because of the doubt and controversy around suicidality, the MNC for treatment is tight, requiring the reported suicidal thought be accompanied by a plan and the means to carry it out if it is to be "covered" by insurance. Parents can and usually do "self pay" for these services when they are denied and appeal their cases later with the MBHO. But the appeal outcomes often reveal medical notes indicating that the underage client was not really "suicidal". Though it makes sense to err on the side of caution in cases of expressed suicidality, the fact remains that being in a psychiatric facility is a very scary ordeal and should be the treatment of last resort.

Serious Mental Illness in Children

I feel compelled in this section to bring up the most vulnerable population that may be overlooked as we waste more money and numerous resources on our ineffective middle monster, damaged care.

More resources need to be applied to children with serious mental illnesses. Mentally ill children are not a large part of the population, but they have the potential to contribute to our society in a large way as adults if they get treatment early. In contrast, if not treated these children spend considerable time disrupting classrooms and exhausting their families and may present later as juvenile delinquents. If not treated, they may become unproductive and even dangerous adults who cost the society more in the long run. Public schools address the challenges of children with less serious disorders through testing and individual treatment plans. These disorders include varying degrees of mental retardation, learning disabilities in reading and math, coordination disorders, communication disorders such as stuttering and the ever popular Attention Deficit Disorders. Of the children's mental illnesses that require more intensive counseling or in some cases a special school environment, autism and Asperger's Disorder come to mind. Under the heading of Pervasive Developmental Disorders (DSM-4-TR,2004), autism and Asperger's are characterized by a profound inability to relate to or interact with others by all conventional standards.   For example, the child may not respond to questions or conversation openers by others or pick up on subtle cues such as body language and facial expression. Their impairments involve language and social communication. As a consequence they have difficulty making friends and maintaining relationships. They may be in trouble at school for disobedience to authority figures. There are other symptoms as well, such as ritualistic (repetitive) behaviors and lack of ability to express themselves appropriately. For example, the autistic child may not be able to ascertain that another child or adult is angry or upset with him and therefore may appear disinterested and defiant.

Autism occurs in 7.2 per 10,000 children according to the last survey done in 1999,- (DVS-IV-TR, 2004), and can be diagnosed between ages two and four. Part of the difficulty is that their symptoms can be found in other childhood disorders such as schizophrenia, mental retardation, hearing and visual disorders, even traumatic brain injury. Therefore it is imperative that parents have their children diagnosed by licensed professionals.

A similar disorder that appears to have no genetic ties but originates with the type of care a child receives is Reactive Attachment Disorder (RAD). Symptoms also include disturbances in interaction with others and appears before the age of 5. Typically, the disorder is noted among children who have been institutionalized without adequate contact with adults. Maternal deprivation, attachment disorder, profound emotional and physical neglect have their effects as early as seven to nine months of age and may be described as a "failure to thrive". Cognitive delays often accompany RAD. RAD manifests in two different types: withdrawn or uninhibited. There is little evidence of the prevalence of this disorder but it is thought to be rare. (DSM-IV-TR, 2004)

Children can also suffer with depression and anxiety, though their symptoms will appear very different from adults. Children who are depressed often act out, and to the non-professional can be perceived as having behavioral problems. Teachers, school counselors and administrators are often ignorant of the impact of depression and bipolar disorder on academic performance. These are as serious as neglect and abuse. Children must be viewed from a holistic stance: academic performance does not exist in a vacuum but is affected by many outside factors.

As an illustration of our ignorance of children's mental disorders I am reminded of a little boy who attended my licensed private preschool many years ago. He was shy and quiet for the most part, with a peculiar habit of repeating everything that was said to him. After working with this child for close to a year I realized he repeated questions and statements from teachers and other children and said nothing else the rest of the time. When I approached his mother to find out what her experience with him at home was, she informed me that he is a "wise guy" who plays that "game" with her all the time even though she punishes him for it. I seriously doubted at the time that this behavior was intentional on the part of the child and insisted she bring him to a specialist such as a child psychiatrist for a complete evaluation. It would be over a year before the mother followed my advice. When she contacted me after his evaluation she presented me with a name for this: echolalia. It was part of a much larger syndrome, Tourette's . (DSM IV-TR, 2004) She thanked me for my persistence and assured me he was undergoing whatever treatment was available at that time. The time was 1990 and I was 30, and as outspoken as I am today.

In conclusion I hope readers will understand that not only have MBHOs squandered money through their bureaucratic waste and mismanagement but that resources and time can be better spent in research and treatment for serious disorders.

The author suspects that the medical community has the same complaint.

Diary Entry: BCBS, 6/19/03

Three Ring Circus

Today was our three way meeting: Desi (current super), Nina (previous super) and moi.. Desi stating I am still making mistakes–an auth not entered, a letter that did not go out...Desi admits they are all "system" mistakes (computer entry mistakes). Nina to me: "We're trying to figure out what the problem is...? Is it the culture, the management or you're maybe having some medical problems...?" (Well, it's all three of you clowns! The so called "culture" is a noisy "ghetto" (their name not mine), the management is unsupportive and sometimes downright mean, the training sucked, the data entry is overwhelming, the stupid system cuts me off after ten minutes of documentation, PAs are restricted) The message is authorize, authorize, authorize and the implication is "Don't think".

...Gotta give this up...God, stay and fight or walk away???

Part III Chap 3

THE MEDICAID MONSTER

Where the Wildest Things Are

As a care manager at Cigna from 2000-2001 I had the dubious honor of managing Medicaid cases. This was my reward after one year of excellent service evidenced by Gold and Platinum Recognition Awards given to me by that company. I was not happy with my new position and I felt somewhat cheated. However, I threw myself into these Medicaid cases just as I had in previous cases. To my dismay, there was little or no oversight and even less opportunity to consult with treating physicians through Medicaid. Children as young as seven were thrown into residential treatment programs for months, and even years without any documented treatment. The facilities appeared to be holding tanks for children who were abused and neglected or just discarded by their parents. While each program required parental participation through family therapy and weekend visits, some of their caretakers knew that the parents of these children were the *real* problems and may not show up at all. "Acting out" behaviors by child patients who had previously participated in treatments that did not work earned admission to the RTC. They were the incorrigibles. Children secluded and far from their homes, they were cared for (so to speak) by a team comprised of social workers trained to work with social ills rather than psychological and medically based ills. There were untrained counselors and doctors who were absent for serving some large MBHO full time instead of keeping office hours at the RTC. How convenient for the MBHO and the State which funded the "treatment". The so called treatment took on the characteristics of baby-sitting, providing some alternative therapies such as art therapy and mountain climbing or other physical activities to help children build social skills and "trust". If asked this author would have committed the parents to the RTC, not the children. Medication treatment and monitoring was rare if it existed at all. Continued stay approval was automatic as dictated by Medicaid and the care manager had little input into the "treatment", such as it was. Weeks would elapse and no MD would see the patient, no trained counselors would conduct sessions with the patient. Months would elapse and children were awarded more continued stays and no visits from family and certainly no "family therapy". The author could not help being flabbergasted by the waste and inefficiency of the State's management of Medicaid and the poor children literally lost in these facilities. Granted, some of the children were a few years away from juvenile court but this is the height of ineptitude. My pay was low, as was my support and any chance of being switched out of this position, because, the manager explained, I was *so good* at this! Without an MD consultant to support my recommendations, I started to feel helpless for the first time as an employee of the MBHO. I was as secluded as the vulnerable young patients were. My education and training were worthless. I had to endure hearing stories of abuse and neglect that were horrific, and I was expected to document all of it without having any impact on it.

Medicaid for Dummies

According to the Centers for Medicaid and Medicare services,

> Medicaid does not provide medical assistance for all
> people with limited incomes and resources. Even under
> the broadest provisions of the Federal statute (except
> for emergency services for certain persons), the
> Medicaid program does not provide health care
> services for everyone. You must qualify for Medicaid.
> Low-income is only one test for Medicaid eligibility.
> There are other established thresholds that vary state
> by state that must also be met.
> (US Dept of Health & Human Services, CMM, n/d.)

Really? Many of you may have thought that Medicaid covered all uninsured children. But the CMM goes on to explain that...

> Your child may be eligible for coverage if he or she is a
> U.S. citizen or a lawfully admitted immigrant, even if you
> are not (however, there is a 5-year limit that applies to
> lawful permanent residents). Eligibility for children is
> based on the child's status, not the parent's. Also, if
> someone else's child lives with you, the child may be
> eligible even if you are not because your income and
> resources will not count for the child.
> (US Dept of Health & Human Services, CMM, n.d.)

To reasonable readers, does it appear that the child's status can be determined outside the family environment? Isn't the child's status dependent upon the parents' or guardian's status? Who's children live in poverty while their parents live above poverty?

My investigation into this monster has uncovered that Medicaid is actually a huge hole where anyone can receive assistance if they meet the loose and subjective requirements poorly explained at this website. Or they can languish indefinitely with poor services or no services. My mind drifts: Bring me your infirmed, your blind, your disabled, your handicapped, your underserved, your downtrodden..... so Medicaid could stomp on them!

> Many groups of people are covered by Medicaid. Even within these groups, though, certain requirements must be met. These may include your age, whether you are pregnant, disabled, blind, or aged; your income and resources (like bank accounts, real property, or other items that can be sold for cash); and whether you are a U.S. citizen or a lawfully admitted immigrant. The rules for counting your income and resources vary from state to state and from group to group. There are special rules for those who live in nursing homes and for disabled children living at home. (US Dept of Health & Human Services, CMM, n.d.)

As stated in an earlier section of this book, Medicaid fills in gaps in coverage for over 40 million low-income Americans. In some cases eligibility requirements can be very strict; one might say they are shrouded in mystery as damaged care has been described. For example, Section 1115 is a waiver to expand eligibility for adults who are neither disabled nor elderly or do not have dependent children. (Overview National CHIP Policy, Children's Health Insurance Program Reauthorization Act,

1997) On the other hand, complex enrollment procedures make it difficult for the very needy to obtain and maintain coverage. Overweight bureaucracy anyone? To worsen matters, in these times of high unemployment Medicaid funds are being cut.

> State Medicaid programs are adversely affected by the confluence of rising unemployment which increases the caseload, decreasing tax revenues during economic downturns, and health care costs that continue to increase several times faster than inflation. Medicaid spending in recent years has outpaced spending growth in other state programs .
> (State Coverage Initiatives, 2008)

In summary, Medicaid needs an overhaul. Rather than adding additional programs such as SCHIP, updated by the Bush Administration (2007), and again by the Obama Administration (2010) which revoked the Bush Administration's update of 2007, etc, we need an equitable and streamlined program to help adults and children who cannot help themselves.

As a child advocate I often wonder if it would not be more expedient to remove children of the poor from their homes and put them in a well run and positive orphanage program while encouraging their parents to get back on their feet. This could motivate parents to make use of the many services for the unemployed including those without job skills or those with language deficiencies (as in non English speaking) and substance abuse issues.

Imagine a kind of rehab for poor families that would include job training, English language and communication skills training and parent training while the children are kept in a safe loving environment. This author once worked for a similar program at the Dallas Child and Guidance Clinic. Parents with charges of child abuse were sent to a Parenting Program while their children were removed to foster care by Child Protective Services. (I do not support foster care unless this program is also overhauled). A condition of getting the children back into the home was that the program had to be completed successfully by the parents. If planned well, this could cost less than pouring money into dysfunctional environments with no hope of future progress for the families.

Diary Entry: BCBS, 8/30/03, Wire Tapping...

Got my first telephone "evaluation"—this is stupid; they haven't figured out that every UR and every facility and every case is going to be treated differently??? How about taking into account the previous conversation with the UR and what information was obtained there??? I prayed at Mass for God to take this from me and make it His. I prayed for the strength to continue on with this job...They sang my favorite hymn, "You are Mine...I called you by name...I will bring you home...."

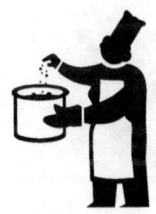

PART IV

AN AMERICAN HEALTH PLAN

Instead of THOU ART MANAGED CARE,
CARE MANAGERS ARE US !

Similar to the managed care for cars model presented in the early pages of this book, imagine this: Consumers go to a local *Policy Store to* purchase a "policy" for behavioral and medical health care. The policy covers the **diagnosis** of all *treatable* conditions that have *proven, successful outcomes,* all necessary tests, and state of the art information about any given ailment. This low cost, customized policy entitles the consumer to a given number of visits to the Policy Store, for a face to face diagnosis with a team of doctors. But treatment is NOT covered; this enables an unbiased diagnosis. The consumer then shops for a doctor (or other providers) who gets paid **directly** by the consumer. The reader is no doubt asking: "How will I afford to pay my doctors for their services!?" Read on: the costs of these services will be significantly lower after this plan is put in place.

A diagnosis of the patient's problem is the first and most important piece of information the consumer needs. Imagine being availed of a team of specialists that can render an *independent* analysis and recommendation addressing the patient's complaint?. The first hallmark of this plan is that consumers receive a *face to face* exam with a doctor or team of doctors without any interference from a third party. The patient receives a coordinated consult from a multi trained team including mental health and medical professionals in the field. This makes the best use of our professionals and our vast cache of medical information. The consumer's complaint is personally addressed and he/she becomes informed about his own condition. The Diagnostic Team is beholden to no one!

Imagine that this policy is customized to fit the individual policyholder and any dependents based on their health care needs and budget. By way of emphasis: the policy parameters are *chosen* by the policyholder; the more health concerns and visits to a doctor the policyholder *estimates* will be needed on an annual basis, the higher the cost of the policy. For example, my policy may include two visits per year for diagnostic services because I have no history of heart disease, cancer or diabetes but I do have a lung disease and/or allergies and/or sinusitis. A well informed "profile" can be built for each individual policyholder. The consumer is now armed with a health profile, vital information about specific health issues and a diagnosis. The author envisions a state-of-the- art center equipped with welcoming and user friendly computers for research and large screen TVs featuring a variety of medical procedures (These are often seen at Vision Clinics where one can view a cataract procedure, etc) Knowledge is power!

Individuality and choice are the second hallmark of this plan. A healthy young policyholder on a limited income may opt for emergency visits only. Flue and food poisoning, a broken ankle or a car accident come to mind as emergencies. Each policy, like the current health care plans, would be renewable and adjustable. Each policy is as individual as each policyholder.
Ingredients that can be added to the new soup mix may include a "major medical" component, flex savings plans, tax credits and an emergency component. Wellness credits that can be traded for other goods and services—maybe even airline miles! This should prove very attractive to consumers. All creative ideas that have been successful in the past can be re-implemented for a comprehensive approach to health care. Some familiar features will sweeten the pot for the consumers.

And the third hallmark of this plan is the use of free markets that flourish with providers competing for consumers. The providers are beholden *only* to the patient! Therefore, they are highly motivated to give the very best of services at the very best cost. Providers will concentrate more on innovation and streamlined delivery to please the consumers. Consumers will determine which providers are "recommended", not some *middle monster (including the government).*! And best of all, providers of all kinds will no longer have to "mess" with damaged care, its paperwork and the extra personnel needed to implement it. Trees will be saved, time will be saved, money will be saved and tempers will be alleviated. In short, the cost of healthcare will go down.

In summary, the American Health Plan features personalization through face to face consultation with doctors, access to unbiased, expert medical opinion and information, choice and free markets leading to lower costs and improved care.

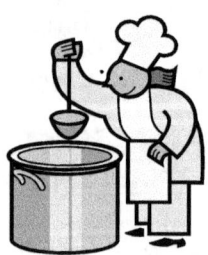

Diary Entry: BCBS, 9/6/03 Breakthrough...

Finally got the antidepressant that works... feeling better....processed with therapist: Magellan does not recognize or reward talent, ingenuity, creativity, problem-solving skills. They are steeped deeply in protocol, political correctness and "corporate speak". They are not interested in emulating the practices of large successful companies such as the Fortune 500– they are short sighted and only interested in profits and current appearances. Otherwise, they would be interested in the some of the ideas I have presented... Thinking of getting out in April 2004 if I can make it till then... I'm overworked, under challenged, and taking orders from people less competent than I am... Go back to Education? Lord, guide me....

PART IV CHAP 1

PEOPLE AND PARADIGMS:

The Haves, The Have Nots and The Will Nots

There are basically three types of individuals regarding their own health care treatment; those who generally *care* for their health, those who generally *don't care* for their health, and those who are *unable* to care for their health. Since this model requires that policyholders be responsible for themselves, it is practical to expect that non compliance will decrease but continue to exist. Non compliance exists for many reasons. In the current plan, there is *no distinction* between those who *will not* care for themselves and those who *cannot* care for themselves. **The author believes that this naive mentality is one of the causes of the demise of the current health care system in America.** The thinking is that the "haves" and the "have nots" must all be accommodated by a system that forces treatment on some and skimps on others in the name of service to an entire population. Where did this mentality come from? It is not an American thought process; it does not illustrate the exceptionalism that is America and its advanced medical and health care portfolio! This is an integral and pertinent discussion that needs to happen among readers and policymakers! As stated earlier, even those who believe that health care can be *forced* upon populations are seriously disappointed when it does not work. One can scrap the history books and simply look around; the one-size-fits-all approach has not worked wherever it has been tried. We are told that droves of patients enter the emergency rooms of our hospitals with serious conditions developed over a period of time, time better spent in preventive care, healthy diet and lifestyle. Droves of these same individuals do not possess a prepaid health care policy, nor can they pay for their treatment. Would anyone deny that when volumes of people utilize a health care system without paying for it that the rest of the population will then *have to pay for it? Or that the alternative is mediocre care for everyone?* This is not "rocket science", as they say. Nor should reasonable individuals plan a health care system around the crazy paradigm that people can be *forced* to care for themselves. A more logical and compassionate understanding of human kind is the acknowledgment that some folks *will refuse* to get treatment for their ills, and then focus our attention instead on those who *cannot* care for themselves but want to. This distinction is essential to understanding <u>An American Health Plan</u>.

The Have Nots

In the author's model, policies are affordable for many more than the 67% who have them now. In addition, the Have Nots are not excluded in <u>An American Health Plan.</u> The plan results in lower costs not only for policies but for visits to treatment providers as well. Hence more of the poor will be able to pay for and participate in the new plan. This said, we will still have a population of individuals who cannot afford the policy or even a visit to a doctor.

Jesus said: "The poor will always be with us". We know that aging and disability can hardly be prevented. Americans need to take full responsibility for these populations, who are *faultless* victims who will indeed always be with us. That the poor will always be with us has been true from the beginning of time, and certainly throughout America's short history. This, despite the solutions tried to eliminate poverty. National Welfare Program, War on Poverty, and a multitude of entitlement programs including Medicare and Medicaid have not improved the conditions of the poor. It is not my intention in this book to insinuate that a free market run health care system will eliminate the poor, but improvements in the overall health care system will trickle down to the Have Nots in ways that improve current access, treatment quality and cost. It is also not my intention to suggest that the poor should not receive our assistance. *I am **not** opposed to a federal or State funded program for the poor in collaboration with faith based and charitable organizations.* I am opposed to waste and fraud; I am opposed to programs that fail to dignify our most vulnerable citizens by separating them from the general population and surrendering them to substandard care. I am opposed to the mentality that all the poor are the same.

Who are the poor? I bring statistics to this section because the poor have been so exploited by our media and politicians for their own purposes that many do not know much about this population at all.

Here are some interesting facts about the poor:
According to the 2008 census numbers as little as 12% of Americans live below the poverty level ($22,000 for a family of 4). *About half of the poor (50%) are elderly.* A significantly smaller group is children (10% of white children, 28% of Hispanic children, 27% of Native Americans and 33% of blacks all live below the poverty level). Are you beginning to get the picture? It is worth repeating: 12% of the American population is poor/. It appears that the elderly and the disabled are our largest vulnerable groups, and children in poor families make up the rest of the 12%.   It can also be presumed that the mentally ill fall into the "disabled" category. Of course *some* or *any* is too many, but we can serve them better than we do currently through Medicaid and Medicare. (US Census, 2008)

More facts from the US Census Bureau: an undeniable relationship exists between education level and earnings; the more education one has the higher the earnings. There is also the obvious connection between how *much* one works and one's earnings. Contrary to popular belief, the reasons people do not work **have least to do with not being able to find a job and more *overwhelmingly* due to having a disability.** It is also not a leap to suggest that minorities such as Hispanic, Native Americans and blacks have the lowest levels of *education* and therefore the lowest *earnings*? But wait, public education is free and available to everyone! The problem of high school dropout rates among Hispanics, Native Americans and blacks needs to be addressed as the origins of this phenomenon are complex and many. Let those dialogues begin rather than passing out expensive band-aids such as free health care for all.

We can address our poor by first accepting that: 1. some number of poor will always be with us, and, 2. that the current programs do not provide compassionate quality treatment for them. Medicare and Medicaid must also be overhauled. We will have to acknowledge that socialism or theocracy or any other form of government will not eliminate the poor. We will have to read our American and world history books to see what attempts have been made *and failed* to eliminate the poor. We will have to define and distinguish the "Have Nots" from the "Will Nots" so that our compassion and efforts are not squandered, but concentrated on those who have legitimate needs, such as the physically and mentally disabled, the elderly and children of the poor. In addition, it is incumbent upon us to establish who among this population have the will and the motivation to follow a health care plan as described in this book.

The Will Nots...

As stated in a previous section, there are those among us who will not take advantage of a *free visit* to a doctor let alone sign on to a health care plan. As a consequence, their illnesses tend to be more serious and they drain health care services and ERs for expensive treatments that everyone else has to pay for. Free health care under the current system is actually available to the Will Nots through hospital ERs. In mental health terms, this is referred to as "enabling". Who are the enablers? Policymakers who think it is kind to force the medical community to service the Will Nots and activists who propose universal health coverage for all Americans are all enablers. Those among us who are kind and generous and compassionate but who fail to distinguish the Have Nots from the Will Nots are enablers.

Who are the "Will Nots"? <u>They are a segment of the poor indeed.</u> What distinguishes them from the *actual* poor, is that they are poor *by choice.* Some are unemployed–by choice; some are uninsured-- by choice; some ignore their health--by choice. Others are uneducated—by choice (since we offer free education in this country) or by neglectful parenting. Lack of education according to the Census Bureau correlates with underemployment and low income. I can attest to this having worked at the Salvation Army with the homeless, unemployed, and domestic violence victims as well as first time drug offenders. The common thread among these groups is that they are under educated and under employed. Some readers may ask: "what came first, the chicken or the egg?" Since high school comes before adulthood, it is most certainly *education*! My opinion aside, there are no statistics on the Will Nots, yet we all know one or two... This is because there is no open discussion about the Will Nots among policymakers. They are simply lumped in with the poor. We do not know how large this "segment of the poor" actually is; we just know it exists. It reminds me of how the entire population must remove its shoes to board a plane because of the actions of one or two thug terrorists! Rather than enable the Will Nots and scrimp on the Have Nots, let's have an open discussion about those among us who are needy by choice.

Some of you are wondering how the "Will Nots" will be identified. You are asking "Why, who among us can make such a judgment?!" Then I ask: Who makes the judgment about identifying the poor or the disabled? Who makes the judgment about special needs children receiving services? Who makes the judgment that the elderly should be shoved and poked to fit into a plan with no choice and poor quality of care? Who makes the judgments about what is fraud and what is medical necessity criteria? If all of these judgments are acceptable, then why not apply a criteria for the population of folks who refuse to care for themselves until it is too late?

And Those In Between

What about the mentally ill? Often we cannot ascertain whether they want care or not. The author has described this population as often "reluctant" to seek help or to recognize their need for it. Theirs are life threatening emergencies which will continue to be routed to the local ER for stabilization, just as surely as the sudden heart attack the dog bites and choking babies will be. The difference for them is that they may be among the designated "disabled", and may certainly qualify for and deserve our assistance.

Natural Consequences

Consider car care again. There are those who take care of their cars, those who don't. There are consequences when one does not take care of one's car. Or, consider purchasing appliances. There are those who buy a warranty and those who don't. Declining the warranty offered with one's appliance purchase has consequences and risks.   Some are willing to bare these consequences, take the risks, and some are not. Most of us want our choices respected no matter what they are and are not surprised too much with the outcomes.

Not caring for one's health has consequences, both to the individual and to the rest of the population.   _People die of untreated illnesses all the_ time. Readers can relate to stories of relatives and friends who refuse to stop smoking, abusing drugs, or any other controllable high risk habit and eventually passed on. Now, the author is not suggesting here that one can control all of one's destiny, but rather that each of us has some choices to make about how we will live. The problem is not always one of _access_ to care, it is often one of _personal choice._ Most of those who seek care are served at the expense of taxpayers, and those who do not come forward are sometimes brought to the ER by others incurring even higher costs to the taxpayer--or just die. This is an undeniable consequence of the current health care "system" in America.

Diary Entry: BCBS, 12/12/03

Though I am swamped and behind, here comes Lucy-she has to meet with me. She is telling me about more computer entry mistakes-she is admitting that the CSRs (formerly Intake Workers) are not screening and correcting the information coming in.... Then the conversation deteriorates to: "If the mistakes don't lessen I will have to write a corrective plan"... That is it, things have finally hit the lowest point. I am telling her that other care managers make the same mistakes and I can prove....Then the icing on the cake-"Todd (the worst UR bar none) is complaining about too many PAs and you know we have this unwritten rule about certain facilities, like Starlight and Sundown that they have a 28 day program and we play along even when patients do not meet medical necessity criteria..." Well, I crack back: Don't expect ME to follow any unwritten rules.. and finally, "Anyone can fix the clinical to sound like someone meets medical necessity criteria..."She just can't help putting her foot in her mouth....And I can't help backing down for fear of losing my job...Told her she should support her CMs instead of backing up the people who complain about them. Praying.... and getting urges to file "harassment" charges—like anyone is going to notices...they've ruined my credibility.

PART IV CHAP 2

MANAGEABLE CARE

The concept of a first stop at the Policy Store to visit the Diagnostic Team is not new. *It is a form of managed care.* It is managed care that is *independent of providing treatment* services and impervious to the incentives of corruption. It is managed care that is not *restricted* care. It is a needed service that informs and guides consumers to make better choices in health care treatment and avoid the high cost of purchasing the wrong treatment or time wasted searching for the right type of provider. It resembles the PCP ("primary care provider") or "Gatekeeper" model, with an "open" gate and without the middle monsters who wished to control the patient's decisions. The Diagnostic Team does not hold the power to *deny* or *assign* treatment; it does not choose the provider or even mandate following its recommendations. It is a *prescription* available to those who seek it. **It is the only service consumers need from a managed care model; it is the *only benefit* to policyholders of a managed care model.** The specialty work of the licensed counselors, (currently, care managers), doctors, nurses and psychologists who can diagnose and recommend treatment and address the medical and psychological concerns of a patient is invaluable to us. Having their services allows patients to manage their own treatment. *An American Health Plan* provides this all important first step without the collusion between managed care and treatment providers. More direct relationships between patients and doctors can flourish. without the hungry mouth of damaged care and all the CEOs that run the industry, oodles of money will be saved. Without the federal government funding, propping up and regulating adult citizens as if they were brain dead, health care can be more accessible to more of us. Inevitably, research will once again become prominant and this nation will return to its rightful place as the providers of the best healthcare in the world.

Diary Entry: BCBS, 10/14/03, Prayers Answered...Again, I gave up my rumination to Him. Today it was announced that the BCBS Team will begin having rounds for each CMs cases...Yes! Accountability! It will become evident now that all my PAs get upheld and that I am reshaping the team and their demands for more auths, more partial step-downs....I will be vindicated. They're asking me to take over all the child cases... this might work! Still, I know I will never be promoted here—I just want it to be bearable.... Thank you God....

Humpty Dumpty

As a consequence of dismantling the humongous and ineffective managed care system, private doctors and other treatment providers will be back in the business of competing for health care consumers instead of barking to the beat of the managed care drummer. The ranks of healthcare providers both medical and behavioral will increase. More competition leads to lower costs and better quality of care. Without the requirements currently placed on healthcare providers, innovation and efficiency will increase. There is no need to strong arm these professionals! Having had years of training and having taken oaths to care for patients, they deserve the opportunity to reach their greatest potential! The improvement in services is a natural consequence of offering people choice through competition. Policyholders will flock to the best doctors and other healthcare personnel who can provide the best treatment, at the lowest cost, in the most comfortable setting, in the shortest period of time. Likewise, providers of treatment will strive to give the best quality of care they can by sharpening their skills. When quality of care improves, policyholders will be healthier and better informed; a nation and its citizenry are more productive. Increased productivity leads to more money to spend on the other ills we face as a society. Competition and free markets saves the day again.

Imagine the freedoms and advantages small and large businesses will reap without the expense of providing health care to employees. No doubt these employers will be able to focus on their company's stated goals. Employees will no longer cling to unsuitable jobs because they need the health care provided to them. Research, advancement, growth, improved services and products will fill their board meeting itineraries instead of reports of the next health care increase or hesitations to hire new employees who will require health care. Attracting the best and brightest personnel, improved retention plans and community contributions will be a significant part of their daily business instead of facing ruination due to employee benefits. No longer will they need a health plan "representative", the middle monster to the middle monster! Thanks to lifting this burden on business, their costs to consumers will also decrease. We all win!

Since the battered providers are no longer saddled with the expense of managed care and the beleaguered employers are no longer oppressed by having to provide healthcare to their employees, both can concentrate on being the best they can be at what they do. Again, this is capitalism and not rocket science; the cost of healthcare will fall and more of the Have Nots will be able to afford it.

When the doctor's bill is $100 instead of $250 plus, more citizens will be able to afford their own healthcare. When hospital rooms come down to $500 per night instead of $5000 per night, healthcare will no longer devastate the middle income families of this nation. When consumers are paying for their own healthcare, they take better care of themselves and avoid the common lifestyle pitfalls that cause some illnesses such as smoking, alcohol abuse and drug abuse, obesity, or skydiving without a parachute. This author's prediction is that health care treatment itself will cost what most consumers pay now for premiums, co-pays and deductibles together in the current system. Work places will experience a rise in efficiency and productivity and workers will enjoy a rise in self esteem and motivation. Employers will be free to hire more employees and pay better salaries without the albatross of providing health care benefits to all of them. Consequently, unemployment will likely *decrease*. When unemployment decreases, still more people will be able to afford their own healthcare costs. As discussed in the Preface section of this book, a different mentality emerges when folks have to be responsible for themselves. Ok, I'll say it: we tend to be wasteful when we receive free stuff! But, fewer people will be left to fend for themselves until they reach the level of serious illness and must admit to the local ER. The local hospitals will get some relief from its staggering budget and overwhelmed ERs and will be able to apply more resources to better quality care. Do you see where this is going?

Counting the Blessings...

Let us summarize the benefits of a consumer driven free market system of healthcare.

1. Policyholders have choice and freedom
2. Quality of health care increases, advances are made
3. Professionals and treatment providers increase in number
4. Competition among professionals means lower costs
5. More individuals can afford to pay for health care
6. Individuals manage their health better
7. Workers become better employees; employers become profitable; savings are passed on to customers.
8. Profitable employers expand and hire more workers
9. Medicaid and Medicare patients have more choices and services
10. Higher employment leads to more consumers, more consumer spending improves the economy.
11. A healthier population leads to more national productivity, paving the way for more innovation
12. A productive nation cares for its citizens, happier citizens make good ministers for the downtrodden.
13. A better nation makes a better neighbor to other countries and more significant contributions to the world!

Diary Entry: BCBS, 11/15/03 Fantasy Interview

I'm imagining my Exit Interview with VP Sue...   I tell her Magellan let me down...I thought it was the company I would grow old with and retire from, no more hunting for the "right place" for me, no more being a "newbie" and frustrated... But no, it had become a company I could no longer respect, a company that makes knee jerk decisions with short term visions that have long term negative consequences, a company long on protocol and political correctness and short on ethics and ingenuity, a company I can add no value to, a company where no one cares about the patients and their own future for that matter...   I hurt so much—I cried and cried...I blamed God then apologized to Him...then asked him for strength, guidance and the self esteem to look for something better...

The Natural Flow of Things

The author's premise for this free market, consumer driven approach to healthcare is that it is consistent with human nature as we have come to know it. Can anyone deny that human beings strive from birth to survive and thrive? To do so is to deny the understanding we have of human nature and our own history. Would anyone argue with the premise that people prefer choice and freedom to being dictated to? Is it surprising to accept that human nature responds positively to challenges to excel? Or that those not challenged *quit trying to excel?* Have we not witnessed the effects of helplessness over one's destiny? Have we not learned that those who contribute less to their own welfare and expect others to do so are often doomed to repeated ineffectiveness? Are these principles not illustrated in history? Free market capitalism is consistent with human nature, which is why it works.

Freedom, Choice and Self Destruction

Non compliance is to be expected in a free society. Rather than trying to "cure" it, a nation should endeavor to *work with it.* Poverty, unemployment and lack of education exists; let us aim to *alleviate it.* The hope to <u>eradicate</u> these conditions, as stated in a previous section is utopian thinking. We live in an unequal and unfair world. Pain, suffering and loss are not divvied up in measured doses and spread throughout the population equally. Likewise, we are not all endowed equally from birth. These are undeniable human truths, not just some "viewpoint" to be debated. Diseases and handicaps are dealt out indiscriminate of a person's worth, value, intelligence or income. Dysfunction, criminalism, anti social and self destructive behaviors have complex origins. They are sometimes byproducts and sometimes precipitants of mental illness. The research on this is *inconclusive.* As discussed in the Preface section of this book, this author knows what it is like to be unemployed and scared, to be uninsured and sick. Most of us want to spare our fellow citizens from this situation. Some believe these ills can be prevented and/or controlled in a socialist, communist or theocratic model of society. I would challenge these believers to find such a society. Some others believe that at the very least the federal government should guarantee (and pay for) healthcare for all citizens. This they believe will eradicate all the pain suffered by those who cannot afford healthcare. Our humanitarian senses are drawn to a "free health care for all" concept initially, but *the vast majority of us won't stand for it in practice!*

It is time to decide where we stand on this history making issue of our times, health care. What we decide will change our society as we know it. Choosing to view healthcare as a "right" rather than a commodity has grave consequences for all of us. Choosing to nationalize any system in a free society is destined to fail if history is our teacher; if it fails humans may not prevail.

Diary Entry: BCBS, 12/01/03, Ghetto Alley

Here comes Carrie, ring leader in the Ghetto, telling me not to bother Desi because he is having a bad day...What the hell are you the Speech Police?! I can't believe I said that—I'm getting sucked into the meanness in the Ghetto, the sarcasm, the backbiting, the "culture" of the alley...

Question: Does good ever win in this world? Scared and helpless—better I should quit than have them fire me... Can't go job hunting—too wiped out from this crazy place...

PART IV CHAP 3
IMPLEMENTATION:

Shopping the Policy Store

So let's review the new terminology in manageable care:

"**Single Payer Plan**"- I'm single, you're single and some of us are heads of a single family. We each pay for our own plan.

"**Public Option**"- We are the public. Most of us will opt to purchase a health care policy; the Will Nots may decline a policy but will be expected to pay for treatment anyway.

"**Preexisting Conditions**"- covered

"**Policy Store**"- a place to buy a health care policy, information and rewards or get a diagnosis for a complaint.

"**Health Care Policy**"- a paid policy that enables consumers to design a package of visits to the Diagnostic Dept for full exam/labs and a diagnosis for their complaint. Does not cover treatment.

"**Insurance Company**"- sells insurance for home, car, etc. No longer in the health care business.

"**Hospital**"—an alternate place to go for treatment with referral by a doctor and for emergencies without referral.

"**Middle Monsters**"—damaged care or the government. Not in the health care business

"Employers"—hire and pay individuals for work. Not in the health care business

"Providers"—facilities, doctors, nurses and other medical or mental health professionals who provide treatment for pay.

The Policy Store would pay for itself through the sale of policies, with one branch for a population of a fixed amount. Rather than call the damaged care company, call for a face to face appointment with the Policy Store nearest you or just walk in. These centers should be spread out so that they are convenient for everyone. A focus on local control and accessibility is crucial. The number of sites will increase as consumer demand increases. Current local clinics can easily transform into this new model. Some clinics already employ the staff needed for the new Policy Store. The benefit of this is that the faces become familiar, comforting and a source of stability for consumers experiencing illness. During the transition consumers will visit the Policy Store when their previous health plan expires to purchase a policy. Still more will visit when they are no longer "covered" as dependents by their parents. Others will be new to choice and individuality, no longer on the government dole drums. And finally, some will choose not to go the Policy Store but to go directly to a provider or the local ER. The author expects that after learning that they will have to self pay for their services that a percentage of the latter population will convert to the American Health Plan because it provides a foundation and education about an individual's health issues.

A visit to the local Policy Store might be a once or twice per year sit down, face to face visit with a Policy Advisor. Policy Advisors may complete a health history (medical and behavioral) and with the consumer's input design a customized Policy. The Advisor is an educator, with charts and statistics, information on the most current medical breakthroughs in a huge database for anyone to come and explore. This local but centralized information database is essential for any society determined to educate consumers about health issues. The author's vision is similar to health related web sites that inform and explain, and even locate providers. Combine this with access to video viewing of procedures as mentioned previously and an inviting learning environment would become a standard at the local Policy Store.

Imagine being able to view a by-pass surgery or a radiation treatment or any other medical procedure of one's choice?! After consulting a with a Policy Advisor, the consumer is better equipped to understand his own health needs to project a number of future visits to the Diagnostic Team for the following one year period. The policyholder will then choose the treatment according to his/her personal wishes (and budget).

In America we currently have all these resources but have never made them centrally and conveniently available to all consumers. Even the new Policy resembles the current health care plan or "policy" purchased from the Insurance Company or an employer, but will be considerably less expensive because the middle monster is eliminated. In addition it is designed for and by the policyholder

For example, the consumer purchases a policy at say, $100 per visit for 5 visits, or $500 for the year. As people age, fewer of these visits would be needed as consumers learn what their health issues actually are. Heart disease and schizophrenia need not be re-diagnosed repeatedly. For those who do not use up all their visits by the end of the policy year, the "roll over" concept can be applied. This is an improvement to the current health savings account in which the consumer loses all their unused (and hard earned) dollars. (The author has always wondered where all this "unused money" goes...) A roll over health savings account is a great idea that can be offered in conjunction with the rest of the new model.

Diary Entry: BCBS, 11/30/03 "Set Up"

They idolize Desi (David)... why can't they see he has lost interest in his team, he hates Magellan, believes his whole problem is about under staffing... What do they know? Only what he tells them—no one monitors this team—no one is accountable here—they are the "non risk", non efficient team... What has he done for this staff?? 1. They are behind the rest of the company and don't even know or care about stuff they are supposed to know, like consulting with docs, shaping facilities, are negative toward other teams, 2. He's out of touch with the rest of the floor and what others have done to improve the process of care management.. Work flow is a problem, work distribution is a problem, the Queue isn't working except to slow things down, his CMs are goofing off for hours and behaving inappropriately for the work place...3. What about Lucy—standing five feet away from me carousing with the ghetto CMs while I'm breaking my back and need help... This team is crumbling! I'm worried about being set up to be fired...God, what is fear and what is paranoia—what is real???

Diagnostic Team: Care Managers R Us

Remember the harassed and bullied care manager working at the undisclosed location that is not in the phonebook, slaving away over faceless cases piled into the antiquated computer program? This trained and educated individual has much to offer as a member of a Diagnostic Team. Joined by nurses, medical doctors, psychiatrists, psychologists, and perhaps neurologists and others, this team takes the place of the "primary care physician". The combination of medical and behavioral professionals means each case receives thorough and coordinated analysis. More than one Diagnostic Team may be needed at a given location. This access to an independent group of trained professionals to determine the diagnosis and the recommended treatment is what is missing in today's managed care. The diagnosticians we have in the present system are either abused managed care professionals or anxious treating providers. In the current system, when the treating provider is also the diagnostician, the patient may need to visit several of them to get a correct diagnosis. Just as everything is perceived as a nail from a hammer's viewpoint, so too each specialist may render a skewed diagnosis closely resembling the specialist's training and experience. What a waste! But if the consumer already had a clear and reliable diagnosis, the treating provider will get to focus on treatment and not maintaining a profitable business or filling out claims forms and phoning the damaged care company for permission to treat a condition that may not meet "medical necessity criteria"!

The Perfect Soup: Services and Perks

The Policy Store is a place I want to see in my town and in everyone else's. As the concept and the word spreads, more consumers will avail themselves of this advantage and profits will follow, supporting its staff and building a better service. But the longer term effect is affordable and efficient health care. And the ultimate effect is a healthier and better informed public. As stated earlier, consumers may opt to go directly to their favorite providers for health services. The mentally ill may still be escorted to the local Emergency Rooms. Many have a few favorite doctors they will re-visit. And still others may need emergency treatment which some doctors may elect to provide. How much more personal is this than the ER at a hospital! One advantage to visiting the Policy Store is that it will be available 24/7 bearing resemblance to a combination of the ER and a local clinic or doctor's practice. This feature can take some of the burden off the hospital ERs. Hospital ER's can then focus on serious accidents and widespread diseases or epidemics. Hospitals can accommodate patients referred to them by doctors.

Let's say I believe I had a minor heart attack but actually had food poisoning? Or maybe I sprained my leg but I thought it was broken. I may need to know my condition in the middle of the night but I may not need treatment in the middle of the night.

Or take a different example: I have no idea what I have but it appears serious and emergent and in need of immediate treatment. A visit to the Diagnostic Team is not indicated in this case as it is too time consuming, therefore I go directly to the doctor or clinic of my choice which offers after hours services, not necessarily a hospital emergency room.

The specialists of the Diagnostic Team should be paid according to the going rates for their field: they should not be esteemed any less than their treating counterparts. They have a special gift for diagnosis. They are timely, they are efficient, they are familiar with the latest research (similar to the PCP), they are available (similar to the ER) and they are impartial (unlike damaged care!). They represent the best in the field. And finally, they do not hold your treatment purse string.

Advantages of a Policy

What is the advantage of having a policy? Caring for one's health can become a behavior rewarded with perks and financial incentives. A policy is not unlike an agreement that the policyholder will take care of his/her and family's health. Going without a policy means the individual sees providers at his/her own risk. They are vulnerable to choosing the wrong provider thereby making treatment more expensive and uncoordinated. How many of us know someone who was passed from doctor to doctor only to discover in the end that their condition is different from originally thought? In the preface of this book, the author tells of a similar "wild goose chase" pursuing a simple diagnosis. Selecting treatment based on one's hunches is expensive and inefficient. Incentives, choice and consequences operate in nature and will prevail in this model as well. Some examples of the benefits follow:

1.Have Policy- Gain Wellness Points – for food, travel, etc

2.Have Policy- Reduce the risk of paying multiple doctors to diagnose a particular illness.

3.Have Policy-Have knowledge with which to shop around

4.Have Policy- Have coordinated care that addresses the whole person, climinating duplication of treatments.

5.Have Policy-Save on treatment, get better care.

This approach for consumers who want information and/or a diagnosis. is time saving and more economical and puts consumers in control. At the same time it is small and personal, local and comfy. Number of desired visits to the Diagnosis Dept determines the scope of the policy not what is offered by your current employer or damaged care. When the policy expires, the policy holder may opt to upgrade, downgrade, renew same or go without a policy. Service is premium and choice reigns.

There are no restrictions regarding "in network", "out of network", "covered" or "non covered" conditions. There are no phone calls to the Insurance company or MCO or MBHO to be "pre-certified". There is no mysterious process of approval or appeal. The patient pays for his/her own treatment. Yes! THE PATIENT PAYS THE PROVIDER DIRECTLY! A new concept: health care paid for by the individual receiving it! The provider of treatment has no phone calls to make on your behalf, no forms to complete or extraneous, wasteful (and costly) paperwork to mess with. I call this: An American Health Plan.

The policyholder who possesses a diagnosis, treatment plan and quote is like the car owner who knows what is wrong with his/her car. Is it not easier to find a mechanic when one knows what the problem is? The author feels more confident asking for a new battery than imitating the noises coming from the car's engine for some mechanic! From this author's perspective, knowing the problem is half the battle.

Paying One's Own Way? Costs Go Down !

The policyholder chooses among providers available in the market place. Some policyholders choose on the basis of cost, some reputations, still others choose by comprehensiveness of the treatment delivered. Some flip a coin. The policyholder pays the provider bill directly. The middle monster is eliminated.

and no longer responsible for determining whether or not treatment is cost effective or medically necessary. The cost effectiveness is determined by what the policyholder wants and can afford. The medical necessity is determined by a team of the best independent specialists in the field and the patient. If the reader has any doubts about the afford ability of paying the doctor or therapist directly, read on.... This model will increase the number of providers because they will not have to hock their lives with the insurance company or damaged care company. They no longer have to hire special staff to wrangle with the multitude of MBHOs and insurance companies to accommodate their patients. They would be more secure again about getting paid; they will focus on providing quality care for the love of medicine and the oldest motive known to mankind: profit! (Ambition is great; it is the ingredient that both fuels and drives our economy! It is the very nature of humankind to strive to thrive!) With more providers and more access to treatments, the cost of healthcare goes down. With an emphasis on wellness and maintaining health through a reward system, the cost of healthcare goes down. Eliminate the middle men (and women), their "Queues", their recorded messages, their CEOs, their plush offices, their alphabet soup, and their reams of paperwork and watch the cost of healthcare go down. This plan makes accessing and receiving healthcare a personal choice and it makes healthcare treatment a commodity to be purchased by consumers. As stated earlier, it capitalizes on human nature. It is a paradigm shift indeed to the damaged care of today, but it is similar to the original managed care concept before the government messed with it.

Incentives for Health Maintenance: Wellness Points

No one is forced to go to the Policy Store, but consumers are incentivized by Wellness Points earned by compliance with recommended treatments and evidence of positive outcomes. An example would be the smoker who uses a non smoking program and is nicotine free for a specified period of time. Exercise, good diet, absence of smoking, substance use limitations, compliance with medications all produce Wellness Points.. For example, an individual with a heart condition has been compliant with medication and scheduled appointments with a cardiologist for a period of time. Reward the patient! Wellness Points can be used to purchase an upgraded policy or if none is needed, food stamps or gas stamps. When a consumer has a policy but has no medical/behavioral complaints, that consumer is rewarded with guaranteed Wellness Points. It's <u>An American Health Plan</u>.

Treatment Compliance?

Any doctor who sees the patient at regularly scheduled visits can affirm a patient's treatment compliance. For example, an internist who prescribes Crestor for a patient with high cholesterol and monitors the cholesterol with periodic blood tests would sufficiently document a patient's compliance. Another example is a therapist who is treating a patient with depression by seeing the patient weekly in coordination with a psychiatrist who is managing the patient's antidepressant medication. Monitoring treatment and freedom of choice are not mutually exclusive in <u>An American Health Plan</u> .

Diary Entry: BCBS,12/08/03, Hanging by a thread..

Cried all night, ruminating about Nina-stealing ideas from care managers to make herself look good but not crediting us, about Lucy and Desi and how incompetent they are, about the new guy who will probably get promoted before I do, about how the CMs snipe at each other in the ghetto, about....being set up to be fired. Getting daily e-mails from Maryanna, monitoring my every move, collecting her documentation. God, is this how I am to go down? The place won't get fixed, and I'll be ruined, and unemployed, without healthcare... I am scared, God.

PART IV CHAP 4
ELEPHANTS IN THE ROOM

Proven Failures

More About Medicaid and Medicare

In an article by Rebecca Palmer (2009), Utah board members came together to discuss the poor state of health care in that state and in the country. Health consumers were invited to present their horror stories and options were discussed for reform. Board members tout non-profit, government run health care while consumers tell of their horror stories with same programs. This was one story:

Tammi Diaz, who received a severe head injury during an automobile-pedestrian crash years ago, told the board and audience that she is stuck in her Medicaid program. Her husband can't make any more money, or she would be kicked off the program and unable to pay for care, she said. And if she makes any money selling the crafts she makes, she'd similarly be kicked off. Diaz could be forced to divorce in order to remain eligible for needed care, she said. Following Diaz's testimony, Rowland and the rest of the Board agreed, "The impact of health insurance policies on the economy is just incredible."

Stories like this one tug at the heart strings. But for every case in which people are shafted out of government programs, there is another (or more) about Medicaid fraud. According to one state's attorney general, Medicaid fraud exists both on the provider and the recipient level. Despite the intricacies of the process for obtaining assistance through Medicaid, health care fraud exits. Some of the ways the provider commits fraud are: "phantom billing" or billing for serviced not provided, "up-coding", or billing for more expensive services than were delivered, providing unnecessary treatments, kickbacks and bribery .(Koster, 2009) In 2003, 46 million people were served under Medicaid to the tune of $278.3 billion dollars, **with 16 billion alone going to administrative costs.** Though payments to providers account for more than half of the government's dole out, fraud is also found with the individual recipients of the government plan. Medicaid recipients can loan out their cards, change their prescriptions on their information files, and claim costs that are unrelated to health care. (CMS, 2009)

> "Experts estimate that abuses of Medicaid eat up at least 10 percent of the program's total cost nationwide—a waste of $30 billion a year. Unscrupulous doctors billing for over 24 hours per day of procedures, phony companies invoicing for phantom services, pharmacists filling

prescriptions for dead patients, home health-care companies demanding payment for treating clients actually in the hospital—on and on the rip-offs go. The cheating is brazen because scam artists have figured out that years of lax oversight have made Medicaid easy plunder."

(Malanga,2006, p 1)

As our population ages, more citizens are heaped into the increasingly limited Medicaid/ Medicare system. According to a Hobbs News-Sun article recently,

"a couple retiring this year needs about a quarter of a million dollars to cover medical expenses, ...a 6.7 percent increase from last year...and the cost is expected to rise". Unfortunately, "Medicare pays about half of the health care costs for current retirees and it could be less very soon" Associated Press, 2009)

There should be no doubt in the readers' minds that both Medicaid and Medicare need to be overhauled. With the new American Health Plan the author's theory is that populations receiving government subsidies for health care can be greatly reduced because many will be able to afford their own policies and services. But there will still be the disabled and elderly who will need assistance. This assistance can come from many sources but will be far less expensive than what it is currently

Returning to the paradigm of the Policy Store, Medicaid and Medicare may continue to exist but on a much smaller and more manageable scale. The elderly poor and chronically ill or disabled, children of the poor would ideally be treated no differently from those who choose to access the Policy Store; individually, compassionately and with plenty of choice. Though the treatment they seek will still require payment to the providers of that treatment, they would receive financial assistance from a combination of tax cuts, charitable organizations and churches in the form of prepaid health care accounts.   But the most important difference under **An American Health Plan,** is that populations who currently receive Medicaid and Medicare will be purged of the "Will Nots"! This points to major reform which requires another book. The crucial point is that health care is not a "right" but a choice for those who have or have not.

Diary Entry: BCBS,12/18/03, Gotcha...
With just 5 months left to my sentence, I have to go now...Another three way meeting, I brought in a witness..."You're making too many mistakes, making the reviewers mad and..." well, they just have to document all of this... I knew it was coming....I better get out-I can't take the pressure..

Dismantling a Behemoth: Ding Dong, The Witch is Dead

Conversion from the old system requires our complete attention and skilled planning . Providers can continue to provide services and clients can continue to receive services – this should remain In tact with few minor changes

One challenge would be redirecting the personnel in the MCOs and MBHOs.   Medical and mental health professionals currently employed by managed care can staff the new Policy Stores.   Some worthy managers, supervisors and Intake workers can be retrained to become Policy Advisors, while the CEOs and claims personnel may have to find other jobs. Personnel now working for large clinics and doctor's offices as insurance reps and liaisons may be redirected to other jobs. Much of the work they do is related to the financial field. PR and marketing folks will be needed to disseminate information about the new system and guide policyholders in new procedures. This will not be a short term endeavor; ongoing education will be needed for this change to succeed. This author envisions a hefty campaign focused on outreach and education. Ample discussion about identifying those consumers who may be left behind should continue to take place along with careful monitoring during the piloting of the new plan. At first, unemployment may spike, but this should level off as the MBHO and MCO employees are recycled. and may be offset by savings in other areas.

Some smaller free standing buildings that now house managed care may be converted into Policy Stores if they are centrally located. More smaller buildings will be needed to insure that the population has equal access. Other larger building now housing MBHOs and MCOs can be eliminated.

Medicare and Medicaid recipients should be phased in first. For the first time in their lives they will receive the local, personal and individualized care they deserve. Instead of receiving checks from the government who usually treats them like cattle, the money can be deposited into individual health savings plan designated for treatments and prescriptions. They may choose the providers they wish for the treatments they need. They will receive more continuity of care. This will be much less expensive than the current system because there will be little if any motivation for fraud and waste.

Funds will be available after dismantling damaged care; states may be able to provide to individuals not on Medicare or Medicaid a onetime only deposit to individual *health savings accounts* to equal a percentage of each consumer's current annual premium plus co-pays. This initial investment will jump start the new system. Savings will be realized from curtailing the current waste and double dipping that has been going on in damaged care. All of these visions are possible with concentrated efforts and good planning.

One idea is to phase in the program by states with similar demographics and doctor availability. This will likely make more sense than implementing a large scale change on the entire population. By piloting and re-evaluating the results in a few states, we can eliminate the "bugs" before passing the plan to all the states. For example, the author is concerned for rural areas with fewer providers and people just making ends meet who do not qualify as "poor".

Through a well thought out campaign to educate the public and commitment from the medical and mental health communities to act as advocates for well-being and good health, implementation has few risks. By retaining the relationships between consumers and their doctors and other providers and taking care of Medicaid and Medicare recipients first, the jolt of a drastic change would be mitigated. When the MCOs and MBHOs are eliminated and Medicaid and Medicare are reconfigured, funds will be available for state and federal government to launch the new system with initial individual investments in health savings accounts.

What to Expect

Here is what the author believes will result:

The healthcare professionals will rise to the challenge of innovation and quality care because they can!

The competition for patients will increase; consumers will be in control: costs of healthcare will decrease!

Capitalism and ingenuity will prevail leading to a more productive nation!

A population will become healthier, stronger, more profitable, more capable of contribution to its society!

Our nation will prosper and we will regain our title as the "shiny city on the hill"!

Diary Entry: Magellan, 12/19/03 Resignation Day...
I'm outa here. Can't take it any more. I can't risk being
fired....I didn't think I could risk being poor—but I guess I just
made that choice....

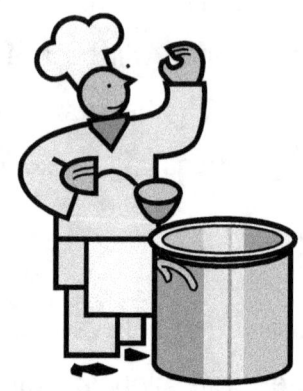

NOTES

At the printing of this book congress had begun debating and developing a new health care plan for America. Finally, after a year, congress passed its new health care bill into law in March 2010. As evidenced by multiple town hall meetings in which democrats were deluged with angry American citizens, the public did not appear to embrace the plan. One of their major complaints was that the bill, now law, contained a "public option" to be offered along with current private health care plans, which could eventually eliminate the private plans and result in government run health care for all. And another strongly opposed feature of the new law is that it mandates that all Americans purchase health care plan or face a fine or jail.

Other complaints about the law included:

1. Abortion may be paid for under this law. (efforts to eliminate this "service" from the new health care plan were voted down by the democrat controlled congress),

2. The potential that "end of life" counseling will be mandated for all citizens age 65 and older with the implication that individuals will be scored for their "value to society" before receiving expensive health care services with Medicare cuts.

3. Privacy issues that can emerge from the centrally located health care data system managed by the government.

4. Management by the government which has already failed at Medicaid, Medicare, Social Security, etc.

But, the most profound complaints came from those who fear incremental socialism:

1. Redistribution of wealth- the probability that the new plan will cost more than the government can afford and will therefore fall on the tax-payers to pay for. These fears were fueled by the lack of clarity about how many non citizens and other "Will Nots" will received health care free of charge

2. The possibility of government "oversight" mitigating the very personal decisions between doctor and patient.

3. The eventual atrophy of competition and choice.

To our credit, the mere hint of socialism does not sell well to Americans, no matter how cleverly it is disguised. Woe to those who attempt to sell us some foreign folly that does not follow our traditional values! Despite the failure of our public schools to produce informed citizens, most Americans have a serious aversion to socialism. Americans are unique in their belief in the following concepts:

Individualism. Because we originally came together as a melting pot of cultures (not to be confused with the cultural pluralism of today) we believe we are equal yet different. One-size-fits all is rejected outright!

Self reliance and self determination. This concept also runs deep within out veins. Why it is what makes our country different from all others. We expect everyone to carry their own weight, unless they are disabled, too young or to old, in which case we are the most generous among nations.

Limited government To Americans this also means limited government intrusion into individual lives.

Equal opportunity. It has always been understood that America affords the most opportunities for unlimited advancement—if one pursues them regardless of race, religion or gender.

The cocky confidence or downright arrogance of Americans perceived by some in foreign countries is an American trademark born of these historic values. We are distinguished by an "internal locus of control" rather than an "external locus of control" in that we believe we can control most of our destiny by the choices we make. Some readers may have experienced the sense of hopelessness and resignation expressed by non Americans and often masquerades as "inner peace". It is anything but.

An unfortunate feature of the current health care law is the pretentiousness and lack of credibility of its salespeople. Hardly anyone can understand its overwhelming thousands of pages written in confounding legalese; the parts we can understand seem suspect. Spokespersons for the plan swear it will cut costs, care for the uncared for, preserve competition and choice, and not impose on taxpayers. But like Damaged Care, the law creates another huge bureaucracy that will require beaucoup feeding and handling by beleaguered taxpayers and will likely impair rather than facilitate the rendering of quality medical services to its members. The government becomes another Middle Monster!

References

Part I Introduction

Cadena, Christine, 2008 Presidential Campaign Platforms: How
      Managed Health Care Issues Impact Us All", 2009 c
      Associated Content, http://www.associatedcontent.com.

Data Points: Health Insurance Coverage...", (2008) US News & World
      Report, 9/12/08.

Lagoe, Ronald, Aspling, Deborah L., Westert, Gert P. (2005) "Current
      and future developments in managed care in the United States
      and implications for Europe," Health Research Policy and
      Systems 2005, 3:4doi: 10, 1186/1405-3-4.
      http://www.health-policy-systems.come/content/3/1/4.\

States' Role in Cost Containment (2008). State Coverage
      Initiatives,Washington,DC,20036.
      http://www.statecoverage.org/node/56

Thorpe, Kenneth E. (2005) "The Rise in Health Care Spending And What
      To Do About It" from Health Affairs, 24, no. 6 (2005): 1436-1445.

"Why are people Uninsured?" (2008) State Coverage Initiatives.
      http://www.statecoverage.org/node113

"Who's Uninsured?" (2007) State Coverage Initiatives, Washington, DC.
      http://www.statecoverage.org/node18

Part I Chap 1

DeNavas-Walt,Carment, Bernadette D. Proctor, and Jessica C. Smith,
U.S. Census Bureau, Current Population Reports, Income, Poverty,
and Health insurance Coverage in the US: 2009, U.S. Government
Printing Office, Washington, DC, 2010

Kongstvedt, Peter J., (2007) Essentials of Managed Health Care, c.
Jones & Bartlett Publishers, Sudbury, MA 01776.
http://www/jbpub.com

Liberman, Aaron & Rotarius, Timothy. (1999) Managed Care Evolution–
Where Did It Come from and Where Is It Going?, Health Care
Manager. 18 (2), c 1999 Aspen Publishers, Inc. p 50-57

Part I Chap 2

Association, May 16-21,2009, San Francisco, CA) reporting on the
results of NCQA annual report for that year.

Bobbitt, L. Bruce, Associate VP, Quality Improvement & Effectiveness,
United Behavioral Health, (2007), The Need for
Behavioral/Medical Integration and Opportunities for Psychology:
A Perspective from Organized Healthcare, p 15, c. 5/5/07, UHC,
Bruce L. Bobbitt @uhc.com

Finch, Ronald, Campbell, Kathryn Phillips & Harbin, Henry, (2006). "An
Employer's Guide to Behavioral Health Services",
NationalBusinessGrouponHealth,
http://www.businessgrouphealth.org/prevention

Frank, Richard G. & Garfield, Rachel L. (2007), Managed Behavioral
Health Care Carve-Outs: Past Performance and Future

Prospects, Annual Review of Public Health, Vol. 28:303-320
(Volume publication date April 2007) First published on line as a
Review in Advance on   November 17, 2006
http://arjournals.annualreviews.org/doi/abs/10.1146/a
nnurev.publhealth.28.021406.144029

Improving Total Health & Well-Being: An Innovative Approach That
Integrates Behavioral Health Across the Health   Care
Continuum, (2006), Open Minds, Sept 2006, p 1

Managed Behavioral Healthcare Organizations, Appendix T, (2001)
Office of Health Care Systems and Financing,   Oct 2001, APA.

Moran, Mark (2004), Health Care Economics, "MCOs still not getting
Mental Health Care Right", Shaping Our Future: Science and
Service (162nd Annual Meeting of the   American Psychiatric

Mulligan,Kate (2002). "California Finds Parity Affordable, But More
Patients forced into Carve outs", p 4., Psychiatric News, June
7,2002, Volume 37, Number 11, c. American Psychiatric
Association

NCQA'sMBHOReportCard,(n.d.), as reported by PsychotherapyFinances
http://hprc.ncq.org/mbho/results.asp

Psychiatric News (2008) American Psychiatric Association
8/01/08, Volume 43, Number 15, p 26.

Rosenbaum, Sara, JD, (2003), "Managed Care Corporate
Failures; An Overview of Bankruptcy and Insurance
Insolvency Procedures", Center for Health Services
Research and Policy, Department of Health Policy, GWU
School of Public Health and Health Services, p1-4

Taub,Carl, (1999), Managed Behavioral Healthcare and Supply   Side
Economics, The Journal of Mental Health Policy and Economics,
1999, 2, 21-28. John Wiley & Sons

Thurston, Jeffrey,M.D. (1996) The Death of Compassion: The
  Endangered Doctor-Patient Relationship, Wrs Publishers,
  Waco, TX 76710

Wilkins, Wallace, (2006), "Managed Behavioral Healthcare Isn't",
  Independent Practitioners, Spring, 2006

Part II Chap 2

Abstract: Influence of the HIPAA Privacy Rule on Healthcare. (2008)
  published byJAMA1/14/2008,Washington,DC.
   http://jama.amaassn.org/cgi/content/abstract/298/18/2164

FindLaw (1975), Erisa and Healthcare Plan Enforcement,
  Employee Rights Center; Wages & Benefits..
   http://employment.findlaw.com

Hellinger, Fred J. & Young, Gary J., (2005). Government, Politics and
  Law. Health Plan Liability and ERISA:The Expanding Scope of
  State Legislation, February 2005, Vol 95, No.2, American
  Journal of Public Health, American Public Health Association

Miller, Tom (2001) Litigate or Regulate, article first published in
  NationalReviewOnline,July3,2001.
  www.cato.org/pub_display.php?pub_id=3963 - 34k - 2001-07-12
  NCQA and Quality Improvement (2003),Training provided
  at Magellan Behavioral Health 4/8/2003. http://www.ncqa.org

Texas Department of Insurance (2005) Texas Insurance Code,
  Title 14,Chap 4201, "Utilization Review and Independent
  Review Agents Subchapter A: General Provisions", p 1-23,
  RetrievedMay7,2010fromhttp://www.tdi.state.tx.us

The Impact of FERPA (Family Educational Rights and Privacy
  Act) and HIPAA on Privacy Protection or health information at
  school: Questions from readers. (2003) The Center for Health

and healthcare in schools, School Based Mental Health
http://www.healthinschools.org/ejournal/2003/privacy.htm
See also:http:www.hrtw.org/tools/laws
See also:http:www.hrtw.org/healthcare/laws
URAC (2001) Overview of URAC, presented at Magellan
Behavioral Health Care Manager Training 7/12/01,
Washington, DC 2005 Current © 2003-2009 ® All Rights
Reserved. http://www.urac.org
US Dept of Health& Human Services (n.d.) Office for Civil Rights-
Health Insurance Portability and Accountability Act of
1996(HIPAA)Washington,DC.http://www.hhs.gov/ocr/hi
paa;http://www.dol.gov/dol/health-plans/portability.htm

Part II Chap 4

First, Michael B., Tasman, Allan, (Editors), DSM-IV-TR Mental
Disorders c. 2004, John Wiley & Sons, Ltd.,
WestSussex,England. p 739-740
Report from Fox News Channel, 2/23/2005
Rampage 'was not a surprise', 4/5/09, Hobbs New Sun, p 28

Part III Chap 2

First, Michael B., and Tasman, Allan,(2004) DSM IV-TR, John   Wiley &
Sons, Ltd., West Sussex, England, p 208
First, Michael B., and Tasman, Allan,(2004) DSM IV-TR, John   Wiley &
Sons, Ltd., West Sussex, England, p 137
First, Michael B., and Tasman, Allan,(2004) DSM IV-TR, John
Wiley & Sons, Ltd., West Sussex, England, pp 255-256
Level of Care Guidelines,(2003), Cigna Behavioral Health

Dallas, TX, 6/16/03

Rudd David M., Ph.D., ABPP. (2004) CEU Workshop: Lives and
Liability: Suicide Risk Assessment, Clinical Management
and Documentation, (5/28/04)

Suicide, Facts At a Glance (2007), Center for Disease Control
and Prevention, National Center for Injury Prevention
and Control (Summer, 2007) http://www.cdc.gov/injury

Part III Chap 3

Children's Health Insurance Program Reauthorization Act, (1997)
Overview National CHIP Policy, retrieved 4/18/2007 from
https://www.cms.gov/

NationalCHIPPolicy/ States' Role in Coverage (2008) State Coverage
Initiatives, retrieved 2/4/2009 from
www.statecoverage.org/node/54

"What is Medicaid" (n.d.) US Dept of Health & Human Services,
updated 4/28/2010. retrieved 5/2/2010 from
http://www.dhhs.state.nc.us/dma/medicaid/index.htm

Part IV Chap 1

U.S. Census Bureau, Current Population Survey, 2008 U.S.
Census Bureau, Annual Social and Economic   Supplement,
2008 http://uscensusbureau.org

Part IV Chap 4

Centers for Medicare and Medicaid Services (CMS),(n.d.),
Overview, last updated 3/09, Baltimore, MD
http://www.cms.hhs.gov/MDFraudAbuseGenInfo/

Koster, Chris (January 2009) Attorney General Missouri, Fraud Control
Unit. http://www.ago.mo.gov/.

Malanga, Steve. (2006) How to Stop Medicaid Fraud, City   Journal,
The Manhattan Institute Spring 2006   http://www.city-
journal.org/html/about_cj.html

Palmer, Rebecca. (2009) "Speakers flay the state of health
insurance", Deseret Morning News. (5/18/09)

$240,000: Retiring today? This is your medical bill, (2009) Fidelity
Investments study reported to Associated Press 3/29/2009

www.ingramcontent.com/pod-product-compliance
Lightning Source LLC
Chambersburg PA
CBHW062129280526
45788CB00001B/103